TABLE OF CONTENTS

TOP 20 TEST TAKING TIPS 4

COLLECTION AND RECORDING OF CLINICAL DATA 5

CHAIRSIDE DENTAL PROCEDURES 25

CHAIRSIDE DENTAL MATERIALS 50

LABORATORY MATERIAL AND 62

PATIENT EDUCATION & ORAL HEALTH MANAGEMENT 67

PREVENTION AND MANAGEMENT OF EMERGENCIES 72

OFFICE MANAGEMENT PROCEDURES 84

RADIOLOGIC IMAGING CONCEPT/PROCESS 94

RADIATION HEALTH 106

PANORAMIC AND SPECIAL IMAGING METHODS 131

LEGAL CONSIDERATIONS 159

SPECIAL PROBLEMS 161

SECRET KEY #1 - TIME IS YOUR GREATEST ENEMY 163

PACE YOURSELF 163

SECRET KEY #2 - GUESSING IS NOT GUESSWORK 163

MONKEYS TAKE THE TEST 163
$5 CHALLENGE 164

SECRET KEY #3 - PRACTICE SMARTER, NOT HARDER 164

SUCCESS STRATEGY 164

SECRET KEY #4 - PREPARE, DON'T PROCRASTINATE 165

SECRET KEY #5 - TEST YOURSELF 165

GENERAL STRATEGIES 166

SPECIAL REPORT: ADDITIONAL BONUS MATERIAL 170

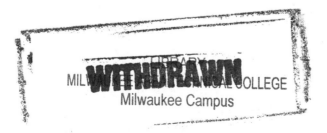

Top 20 Test Taking Tips

1. Carefully follow all the test registration procedures
2. Know the test directions, duration, topics, question types, how many questions
3. Setup a flexible study schedule at least 3-4 weeks before test day
4. Study during the time of day you are most alert, relaxed, and stress free
5. Maximize your learning style; visual learner use visual study aids, auditory learner use auditory study aids
6. Focus on your weakest knowledge base
7. Find a study partner to review with and help clarify questions
8. Practice, practice, practice
9. Get a good night's sleep; don't try to cram the night before the test
10. Eat a well balanced meal
11. Know the exact physical location of the testing site; drive the route to the site prior to test day
12. Bring a set of ear plugs; the testing center could be noisy
13. Wear comfortable, loose fitting, layered clothing to the testing center; prepare for it to be either cold or hot during the test
14. Bring at least 2 current forms of ID to the testing center
15. Arrive to the test early; be prepared to wait and be patient
16. Eliminate the obviously wrong answer choices, then guess the first remaining choice
17. Pace yourself; don't rush, but keep working and move on if you get stuck
18. Maintain a positive attitude even if the test is going poorly
19. Keep your first answer unless you are positive it is wrong
20. Check your work, don't make a careless mistake

Collection and Recording of Clinical Data

Patient Records

A patient record is a legal document containing pertinent information related to the individual and his or her care. Retain it at least seven years from the last visit and keep it confidential. On the left, attach the Registration Form for demographics, such as: Patient name; address; phone numbers; employer; spousal or parental information; payer; insurance, if any [photocopy the insurance card]; and chief complaint. On the right side, attach a Medical History, including: Prescription, over-the-counter, and street drugs; exposure to radiation and toxins; medical conditions (e.g., diabetes, epilepsy, pregnancy, bleeding disorders, or rheumatic fever); allergies marked with brightly-colored alert stickers; and height and weight to calculate anesthetic dose. The dentist authorizes the Dental History form. The patient or guardian signs and dates Consent to Treatment and Release of Information forms, for legal coverage and continuity of care. Keep the patient record in reverse chronological order, with the most recent treatment record on top and the oldest at the bottom.

If your patient has any conditions that require the dentist to consult with the physician, then ask your patient to sign a Release of Information form. Before subsequent visits, ask your patient's doctor to complete a Medical History update form. Include laboratory reports for communicable diseases. The diseases of concern are hepatitis and human immunodeficiency virus (HIV/AIDS). Give your patient (or his/her guardian) a written description of the right to privacy under the Health Insurance Portability and Accountability Act (HIPAA).

Keep these signed forms for at least 7 years from the last visit. Document the examination, dental charting, and oral radiography. The dentist reports suspicious lesions or other medical conditions (e.g., suspected heart disease) back to the physician.

Vital Signs

Explain to the patient what you are going to do. Tell your patient not to speak because talking increases BP and decreases temp. Place a clean oral digital thermometer under the patient's tongue. Respiration rate indicates efficiency of oxygen intake and carbon dioxide output. Watch your patient's chest rise and fall. One respiration consists of an inhalation followed by an exhalation. Count respirations for 1 minute while holding the radial pulse (inner wrist on thumb side) with your fingertips, so the patient does not hold his/her breath. Do not feel a pulse with your thumb. Normal adult white male results are: Resp 16 to 20 bpm; pulse 60 to 80 bpm; temperature 98.6°F (37°C). Record a baseline at the preliminary exam. Update TPR at subsequent visits. Document immediately, before the visit concludes. If the patient has no arms or you cannot feel the radial pulse, then feel one of these pulses: Carotid (neck groove beside trachea), brachial (antecubitum below elbow bend), or temporal (depression between eyebrow and ear).

Blood Pressure

Blood pressure (BP) is controlled by the hypothalamus, medulla oblongata, and kidney. Pain, exercise, and fear increase blood pressure. Use either a stethoscope and a sphygmomanometer or an automated BP clip to measure BP. A thin adult needs a pediatric cuff. Use a thigh cuff on an obese patient's arm. A normal adult white male's BP is 120/80 mm/Hg. Small women and children have lower blood pressures. Elders have higher blood pressure. Hypotension (low blood pressure) is below 90/50 mm/Hg.

Hypotension leads to dizziness and fainting. Hypertension (high blood pressure) is above 140/90 mm/Hg. Hypertension leads to stroke and heart disease. The first Korotkoff sound you hear ("lup") is the systole, when the heart contracts to pump oxygenated blood to the arteries from the left chamber of the heart. The second sound ("dup") is the diastole, when the heart relaxes as its right side fills with blood for subsequent oxygenation. BP is the ratio of systolic to diastolic pressure.

Seat your patient (standing elevates BP). Explain what you will do. Extend your patient's arm at heart level. Palpate the brachial artery (inner forearm) for pulse rate. Add 40 to the pulse rate to determine the inflation level for your sphygmomanometer, e.g., a pulse rate of 80 beats a minute means inflate to 120 mm of mercury (Hg). Wrap the sphygmomanometer cuff snugly around your patient's arm 1 inch above the antecubitum (elbow bend). Place the stethoscope bell or diaphragm over the brachial artery. Attach the stethoscope earpieces to your ears. Close the valve. Pump the rubber bulb with your other hand to inflate the cuff rapidly. Listen through the stethoscope while gradually releasing the valve. The initial "lup" is the systolic pressure you record in the patient's chart. Note when the Korotkoff sounds cease. Record the last "dup" sound as the diastolic pressure, e.g., 120/80 mm/Hg. Open the valve to release air. Deflate the cuff quickly to minimize discomfort. Disinfect your earpieces with alcohol wipes afterwards.

Vital Signs

Temperature:
Ideal 98.6°F (37°C) •Normal Range 97.8°F (36.5°C)— 99°F (37.2°C); lowest in the morning.
Hypothermia <95°F (<35°C) from cold exposure or antipyretics.
Pyrexia >98.6°F oral or >99.8°F rectal; use Tylenol for children and Aspirin for adults. • Hyperpyrexia 107.6°F (>42°C); use cold packs.

Pulse:
Normal adult 60—100 beats/min. with a normal sinus rhythm. • Females beat faster than males.
Children beat faster (90 to 120 and neonates 144 beats/min.).
>100 bpm in adults is tachycardia.
<50 bpm in adults is bradycardia. Abnormal rhythm is arrhythmia.

Respiration:
Normal adult 12—20 per min.
Children breathe faster (neonates 30—60 per min.).

Blood Pressure:
Upper normal adult 120/80 mm/Hg
Hypertension 140/90 mm/Hg • Hypotension 90/50 mm/Hg

Pain*:
Pain absent • Responsive to pain stimulus
* Optional, used to monitor patient during procedure and when the patient recovers from anesthesia

Respiration rates depend on the patient's age, pain, level of consciousness, and health status. A healthy adult breathes between 10 to 20 breaths a minute. A child breathes 18 to 30 breaths per minute. A newborn breathes 30 to 60 times per minute. Unusually fast breathing when at rest is tachypnea. Unusually slow breathing when at rest is bradypnea. Difficult breathing is dyspnea. Asthmatics and congestive heart failure patients breathe comfortably only when sitting erect, which is orthopnea. You should not hear wheezing, crackles, rales, rhonchi, or stridor.

Normal adult systolic BP is 100 to 140 mm/Hg. Normal adult diastolic BP is 60 to 90 mm/Hg. Normal values are based on young Caucasian males. High blood pressure is hypertension, a BP exceeding 140/90 mm/Hg. Hypertension indicates the heart is working abnormally hard, especially if the diastolic reading is high, and is likely enlarged (hypertrophied). Low blood pressure is hypotension, a BP below 90/50 mm/Hg. Your hypotensive patient may faint.

External Evaluation

Scrutinize your patient discreetly as he/she enters the room for indicators of abuse, nutrition issues, poor health, and aging. Focus on these issues that impact dental or orthodontic care: Exaggerated facial asymmetry; swelling (edema); speech problems; abnormal lip smacking; mouth breathing; and thumb sucking. Examine the lips for cracking or parching from dry mouth (xerostomia), which indicates underlying disease (e.g., thrush, vitamin deficiency, hypothyroidism, autoimmune diseases, or psychiatric drug use). Examine the smile line where the lips meet, the peripheral vermillion borderline, and the lip corners or commissures. Ask your patient to close his/her lips. Palpate the mandible and external floor of the mouth externally. Ask your patient to turn his/her head to the side. Feel the cervical lymph nodes between the ear and collarbone. To inspect your patient's temporomandibular joint (TMJ) externally, sit behind the patient. Palpate the tragus in front of the ear as the patient opens and closes his/her mouth. Listen for clicking (crepitus). Watch for snagging. Ask the patient if he/she feels pain.

Internal Evaluation

A certified dental or orthodontic assistant can legally perform both the external and internal clinical evaluation in most states. After you examine your patient is extraorally, perform an internal oral examination. Note mouth wounds, abscessed teeth, and abnormal mucosa colorations. Hold the mandible in one hand. Palpate the underside of the tongue and the floor of the mouth. Stand behind the patient. Examine the oral mucosa and frenum (fold) by pulling the lips outward. Use a mouth mirror to inspect the buccal (cheek) area and the tongue. Use gauze to pull the tongue to the side and upward for better vision. Instruct your patient to say "ah". Inspect the entrance to the throat and the oropharynx. In addition, the dentist uses a hand instrument to prod the hard surface of every tooth, and the assistant notes any findings in the patient's record.

Charting

Tooth diagrams are either anatomic or geometric. An anatomic diagram has pictures that look like real teeth, including the roots. A geometric diagram uses divided circles to represent each tooth. The circle's divisions signify different tooth surfaces. Each chart has positions for all 16 upper and 16 lower teeth.

Several different numbering systems may be used. The most common in the USA is the Universal/National System. Other countries use the International Standards Organization System more often. The teeth are shown as if one is looking into the patient's mouth. Indicate completed dental treatments in either blue or black on the chart. Note newly detected or incomplete treatments in red. Use Black's classification system to mark cavities (caries) on the diagram as Classes I to VI. Dental offices may use a variety of symbols or short forms to describe conditions or materials used in the patient's mouth. Ask your office manager for a copy of acceptable abbreviations to avoid confusion.

Basic Charting Terms

Some basic charting terms that are descriptive include:
- Abscess - a deep, limited, infected pocket filled with pus

- Diastema - the gap between two teeth, usually used to describe that between maxillary central incisors

- Drifting - movement of tooth position to occupy spaces formed by removal of another, also called over eruption

- Incipient - areas of developing decay where enamel is still intact, appearance is chalky due to initiation of decalcification

- Mobility - movement of a tooth within the socket quantified in millimeters; generally results from trauma or periodontal disease.

- Periodontal pocket - excessive space (more than 3 mm) in a gum sulcus, due to periodontal disease

- Overhang - presence of too much restorative material

Basic charting terms referring to completed or suggested dental work include:
- Bridge - a prosthesis that replaces missing teeth, held in place on attaching sides (abutments), or sometimes just one side (a cantilever bridge). The middle area is termed the pontic.

- Crown – permanent, custom-made or manufactured temporary tooth covers. Crowns are available in a variety of materials and combinations, including gold, porcelain, stainless steel, and plastic. A crown covers either the full tooth or ¾ of the tooth.

- Denture - a complete (full arch) or partial set of artificial teeth attached to a plate.

- Restoration - materials used to fill caries or replace missing tooth structure, including silver amalgams, composite resins, and gold.

- Root canal - a procedure in which the dentist removes the tooth pulp and replaces it with a filling material.

- Sealant - a resin used to seal pits and fissures in the tooth enamel to deter decay.

- Veneer - a thin material bonded only to the facial aspect of the tooth, usually for cosmetic improvement.

Charting Symbols

Indicate future dental work in red on a chart. Indicate completed dental work in blue. Place an "X" through missing teeth on the chart. If all the teeth in an arch are missing, encircle and place an "X" over it. Draw supernumerary (extra) teeth on the chart. Show drifting or overerupted teeth by drawing arrows in the direction of the drift. Circle impacted or unerupted teeth. Place a red slash through teeth requiring extraction. Indicate diastema with two vertical lines at the gap. Show tooth rotation with a directional arrow on the side. Indicate mobility with two small lines. Draw jagged lines to indicate tooth or root fracture. If a tooth needs a root canal, draw vertical red lines through it. If the root canal procedure has already been performed, draw blue vertical lines through it. Show gingival recession or furcation involvement with wavy lines and dots. A small red circle drawn near the root indicates an abscess. Arrows between roots indicate periodontal pockets.

Dental Caries

Dental caries (cavities) are classified from Class I to Class VI based on the teeth and surfaces they are formed in. Classes I to V were described by a pioneer in the field of dentistry, G. V. Black, and Class VI was included later. They are:
- Class I - developmental caries in pits and fissures, including occlusal surfaces of back teeth, buccal or lingual pits on molars, and lingual pits on maxillary incisors. Restore with tooth-colored composite resins.

- Class II - cavities on proximal surfaces of premolars or molars. Restore with tooth-colored resins, silver amalgam, gold or porcelain.

- Class III - cavities on interproximal surfaces of incisors or canines. Restore with composite resins.

- Class IV - similar to Class III except incisal edge is also involved. Restored with composites, and if considerably decayed, porcelain crowns.

- Class V - caries only near the gum line on either facial or lingual surface. Restore with composites for front teeth and silver amalgam for posterior teeth

- Class VI - cavities on occlusal or incisal surfaces formed by erosion. Various restoration materials are appropriate.

Cavities are charted in terms of whether they involved single, two, three, or more surfaces that have been or need to be restored. A simple cavity restoration involves only a single surface. Simple cavity restorations are described by a letter standing for the surface involved: I (incisal); M (mesial); D (distal); B (buccal); O (occlusal) or F (facial). Compound or two-surface restorations use a combination of two letters that illustrate the two facades involved. Thus, typical compound cavity restorations are described as: OB (occlusobuccal); MO (mesio-occlusal); MI (mesio-incisal); DO (disto-occlusal); DI (disto-incisal); DL (disto-lingual); or LI (lingual-incisal). Complex cavity restorations involve at least three surfaces and the abbreviations for them incorporate all facades involved, for example MOD for mesio-occluso-distal.

Red indicates caries that have not yet been restored; blue indicates caries that were restored. Either fill in the affected surface on the chart, or encircle it with the appropriate color. Chart amalgam restorations by both outlining and filling in. Show composites with outlining only. Indicate recurrent decay of previously restored teeth by outlining the existing restoration in red. For enamel sealants that have been used to deter decay, place an "S" over the area. Temporary restorations are indicated with blue circles. For crowns, draw diagonal lines across the whole area involved if gold, or encircle if porcelain. For fixed bridges, draw an "X" through the root(s) of missing teeth; the area for the bridge is either outlined (porcelain) or indicated by diagonal lines (gold). Show a Maryland bridge, which has wings on the pontic, with curves. Indicate veneers by outlining. For dentures, place "X"s over all involved root areas, and show the corresponding crown areas by either a large circle (full) or dotted lines (partial).

Numbering Systems

The Universal/National System is sanctioned by the American Dental Association and is the most common system used to number teeth in the United States. Children's primary teeth are lettered from A to J in the maxilla (upper jaw) from the right second molar to the left second molar. Children's mandibular (lower jaw) teeth are lettered from K to T starting with the left second molar and ending with the right second molar. Adults' permanent teeth are designated numbers from 1 to 32. Number 1 starts on the maxilla at the upper right third molar, and proceeds consecutively along the top to tooth #16 on the upper left third molar. Numbering of the lower teeth starts on the mandible at the left third molar as tooth #17 and ends at tooth #32 or the lower-right third molar.

Most foreign countries use the International Standards Organization System/Federation Dentaire Internationale (ISO/FDI). Two digits identify each tooth: The first is the quadrant and the second is the tooth. Start numbering in the center of the mouth for

- 9 -

adults and children. The first digit 1 is the adult's right maxillary quadrant; 2 is left maxillary; 3 is left mandibular; and 4 is right mandibular. The second digit for permanent teeth in each adult quadrant runs from 1 to 8, starting at the incisors. Number children's quadrants from 5 to 8 for primary teeth. Children's second digits extend from 1 to 5 because they have fewer teeth. Pronounce digits separately, e.g., "One one", rather than "Eleven".

The UK uses Palmer Notation (Military System). Bracket symbols indicate the quadrant. The digit, representing the tooth, proceeds from the center. Number permanent teeth from 1 to 8. Number primary teeth from A to E.

Adult Universal Numbering System

In this system: Tooth number 1 is the tooth farthest back on the right side of your mouth in the upper (maxillary) jaw.
Numbering continues along your upper teeth toward the front and across to the tooth farthest back on the top left side (which is number 16).
The numbers continue by dropping down to the lower (mandibular) jaw. Number 17 is the tooth farthest back on the left side of your mouth on the bottom.
Numbering continues again toward the front and across to the tooth farthest back on the bottom right side of your mouth (which is number 32).

Adult Palmer Notation Method

In this system, the mouth is divided into four sections called quadrants. The numbers 1 through 8 and a unique symbol are used to identify the teeth in each quadrant. The numbering runs from the center of the mouth to the back.

In the upper right section of the mouth, for example, tooth number 1 is the incisor (flat, front tooth) just to the right of the center of the mouth. The numbers continue to the right

and back to tooth number 8, which is the wisdom tooth (third molar.)

The numbers sit inside an L-shaped symbol used to identify the quadrant. The "L" is right side up for the teeth in the upper right. The teeth in the upper left use a backward "L." For the bottom quadrants, the "L" is upside-down. The quadrants may also be identified by letters, such as "UR" or "URQ" for the upper right quadrant.

Dental Arches and Quadrants

Dentition is the normal arrangement of teeth in the mouth. Teeth grow in one of two dental arches. Teeth set into the maxilla (upper jawbone) comprise the maxillary arch, which is affixed to the skull and has no flexible sideways movement. Teeth set in the mandible (lower jawbone) comprise the mandibular arch, which is flexible and can move sideways and up and down. Adjoining teeth that are correctly positioned touch each other. Maxillary arch teeth contact and slightly overlap those in the mandibular arch when the patient closes his/her mouth.

Dental quadrants are areas of dentition defined by the arch they are in (to the right or left side of the midline of the face). Thus, there are four dental quadrants: Maxillary right quadrant, maxillary left quadrant, mandibular right quadrant and mandibular left quadrant. The primary or deciduous teeth grown initially by children number 20, so there are 5 teeth in each quadrant. There are 32 permanent teeth developed in adolescence, with 8 in each quadrant.

Tooth Function

There are 20 deciduous teeth (10 in each arch, 5 in each quadrant). Starting at the midline and extending backwards, each quadrant contains: (1) central incisor (cutter); (2) lateral incisor (cutter); (3) canine or cuspid (tearer); (4) first molar (grinder); and (5) second molar (grinder).

Thirty-two permanent teeth (16 per arch, 8 per quadrant) function similarly to primary teeth. The permanent teeth in each quadrant, extending from the midline to the back of each arch, are: (1) central incisor; (2) lateral incisor; (3) canine; (4) first premolar; (5) second premolar (bicuspids choppers); (6) first molar; (7) second molar; and (8) third molar (grinder). The anterior teeth in the front of deciduous and permanent dentition are the central and lateral incisors and canines. Anterior teeth have single roots and a distinct incisal edge. Posterior teeth, behind the anterior teeth, have more than one root and cusp (grinding surface).

Primary Teeth

Children's deciduous or primary teeth begin erupting around four to six months of age. Most children have a complete set of primary teeth by 32 months of age. The eruption schedule is similar for both the maxillary and mandibular arch. Central incisors erupt first, followed by the lateral incisors, the first molars, the canines, and lastly the second molars. Primary teeth are shed from the oral cavity or exfoliated in approximately the same order. Exfoliation generally starts at age 6 to 7 years, beginning with the central incisor. Exfoliation should be complete by 10 to 12 years of age. The canines and second molars shed last.

Permanent Teeth

From about age 6 to 12 years, a child has mixed dentition. Permanent teeth begin to erupt during this period before all primary teeth are shed. The permanent teeth that eventually replace the deciduous central incisors, lateral incisors, and canines are succedaneous (they succeed deciduous teeth). Molars are not succedaneous. The first molars are generally the first permanent teeth to come into both arches at about age 6 to 7 years, followed by the central incisors and lateral incisors. The other teeth may come in differently for the two arches. The second and third molars are the last teeth to appear (usually at ages 13 and 21, respectively).

Tooth Surfaces

Each tooth has:
A crown enclosed by enamel
A root faced with a thin layer of bony tissue called cementum
A cervical line (the cementoenamel junction) dividing the two
Anatomical describes the actual covering material of crowns and roots. Clinical refers to the visible portion of the crown and root. Anterior teeth have 5 crown surfaces: (1) mesial, facing the midline; (2) distal, facing away from the midline; (3) labial, exterior opposite the lips; (4) lingual or palatal, interior facing the tongue; and (5) incisal or cutting edge. Posterior teeth also have five coronal surfaces: (1) mesial; (2) distal; (3) lingual; (4) buccal, exterior toward the cheek; and (5) occlusal, the top chewing surface. Another term for labial or buccal surfaces is facial. Surfaces can be convex (curving outward), or concave (curving inward), or flat. Any combination of surfaces can be found on the same tooth.

Anatomical Landmarks

Anatomical Landmarks of Teeth
Bifurcation or trifurcation: 2 or 3 roots emerge from the tooth's main trunk. The dividing spot is the furcation.
Grooves or depressions: 3 types: Buccal grooves, developmental grooves on the occlusal surface; and supplemental grooves emanating from the developmental type. Fissures are imperfectly united developmental grooves. Pits are areas where fissures meet.
Ridges: Elevated sections of enamel. 4 types: marginal, oblique, transverse and triangular. Only marginal ridges are found on anterior teeth. All 4 types are observed on molars.
Fossa: Relatively superficial rounded or angular depressions
Apex: At or near the terminus of the root; the apical foramen is an opening at the apex

through which nerves and blood vessels come into the tooth.

Cusp: Mounds on the crown; most molars have multiple cusps. First molars may also have a fifth cusp on the mesial lingual surface, known as the Cusp of Carabelli. Lobes are united partitions that form teeth (usually equivalent to cusps for molars).

Cingulum: Convex space on lingual surface of front teeth

Mamelons: 3 protuberances on incisal edge of new central incisors

Anterior Maxillary Teeth

Maxillary incisors have sharp incisal edges but no cusps. They have single roots up to twice the length of their crowns. The maxillary central incisors near the midline are slightly larger (both crown and root) than the adjacent maxillary lateral incisors. When central incisors initially erupt, they display three bumps on the incisal surface, called mamelons, which wear down to a flat edge. Incisors have imbrications, or faint overlapping lines and developmental depressions, on the labial surface near the gums. The labial surface of the crown is convex, while the lingual side is concave. Incisors are essential for producing certain speech sounds. Maxillary lateral incisors often vary from the expected. The maxillary canines (cuspids) have the longest roots in the maxillary arch, making them the most secure. The labial surface of the crown is convex with a vertical ridge. The incisal edge ends in a tip. The lingual side has two hollow fossae, separated by ridges. Canines contain more dentin (calcium-containing material) below the enamel, making canines darker than incisors.

Posterior Maxillary Teeth

Maxillary first and second premolars (bicuspids) are posterior to the canines. Premolars have crowns with two cusps. The facial cusp is larger than the lingual cusp. The difference is more pronounced in the first premolar. Maxillary first premolars have two

bifurcated roots, whereas maxillary second premolars have single roots. Proceeding posteriorly are the maxillary first molars, which are almost square and have five cusps: Mesio-buccal, disto-buccal, mesio-lingual, disto-lingual, and the cusp of Carabelli on the mesio-lingual cusp. There is a buccal groove between the mesio-buccal and disto-buccal cusps, and buccal and lingual pits, a central fossa, and oblique and transverse ridges. Maxillary first molars have trifurcated roots. Maxillary second molars are slightly smaller and have only four cusps (minus the cusp of Carabelli); they have trifurcated roots. Maxillary third molars are slighter than the second molars and have more grooves on the occlusal surface. Their root structure varies. Third molars may be absent or fail to erupt, requiring removal.

Anterior Mandibular Teeth

Contrary to dentition in the maxillary arch, the mandibular central incisor is smaller than the adjoining lateral incisor. Mandibular central incisors have single, very straight, pointed roots. The crowns are very slender and sharp at the edge. Initial mamelons wear off. Mandibular central incisors have convex labial and concave lingual surfaces and a cingulum. The only differences in the lateral incisors are larger crowns, with relatively smaller distal sides, and smaller single roots that may have concave surfaces. The mandibular canines (bicuspids) have single roots with deep depressions; they may be shorter than those of the maxillary canines in the upper arch. The crowns of mandibular canines have steeping sloping distal cusps and smaller mesial cusps.

Posterior Mandibular Teeth

The mandibular first premolar (bicuspid) has two cusps on the crown: A prominent buccal cusp and a smaller lingual cusp, with an occlusal groove between. There are mesial, distal, and transverse ridges. Mandibular first premolars have short, single, straight roots. The mandibular second premolar has up to three short lingual cusps and one buccal cusp. Three grooves and ridges are on the occlusal surface. Mandibular second premolars have one distally angled root. The mandibular first molars are the biggest teeth. They have five cusps, meeting on the occlusal face in a central fossa, with grooves in between cusps. The crown is concave on the mesial side but straight distally. This pattern reflects in the two root structures (mesial and distal). The mesial root has two separate pulp canals. The mandibular second molar is smaller than the first, with four cusps meeting on the occlusal surface, and buccal and lingual grooves that terminate in pits. Second molars usually have bifurcated roots. Mandibular third molars are smaller, with multiple roots and furrowed surfaces.

Deciduous Maxillary Teeth

Deciduous (primary) teeth have relatively long roots compared to their crowns, more prominent cervical ridges, and are very white, due to thin enamel and dentin, but more pulp). Deciduous teeth are smaller than permanent teeth. Maxillary deciduous central incisors have distinct cervical lines, are wider than their height, have no mamelons, and their labial sides are convex. Maxillary deciduous lateral incisors are smaller, longer, and more curved than central incisors. Maxillary deciduous canines (cuspids) have pointed incisal rims, ridges on the mesial and distal sides, and prominent cingula. Maxillary deciduous cuspid roots are more elongated than the incisors. All of these anterior teeth have single roots. The maxillary deciduous first molars have four cusps, transverse and oblique ridges, and three roots. The mesio-lingual cusp is the most prominent. Second molars have four or five main cusps, and three widely separated roots.

Deciduous Mandibular Teeth

The mandibular deciduous central incisor is very similar to its permanent replacement, except its crown is wider and both lingual and labial surfaces are curved, while the sides are flat. The mandibular deciduous lateral incisors are slightly longer and broader than the central incisors; they have a prominent cingulum, distal and mesial ridges, and a deeper fossa. Their roots bend distally at the bottom. Mandibular deciduous canines have smaller roots and less prominent crown ridges than their maxillary counterparts. Mandibular deciduous incisors and canines have single roots. The mandibular deciduous first molars have four cusps (mesio-buccal is the biggest), relatively long buccal facades, and bifurcated roots on the mesial and distal sides. Mandibular deciduous second molars look like permanent mandibular first molars, but are smaller. The mesio-buccal and disto-buccal cusps are about the same size. Mandibular deciduous second molars have two roots; the mesial root is bigger than the distal.

Oral Inflammation

Inflammation is the body's reaction to infection, allergy, or injury. Inflammation is characterized by redness, heat, swelling, and pain. Inflammation occurs because an injury, allergy, or disease causes immune cells to release histamine into the area. Histamine increases blood flow, manifesting as redness and heat. Histamine makes vessels leaky. Excess blood seeps from the capillaries into surrounding tissues, causing distension. Nearby nerve receptors register inflammation as pain. White blood cells (leukocytes) are recruited to the site to kill microorganisms. Fibrous connective tissue surrounds the area in a web. Be attuned to the signs and symptoms of inflammation because they represent an underlying disease process. Oral inflammation can be observed as a variety of lesions on the mucosal surface.

Oral Lesions

Shallow lesions that appear on the surface of the oral mucosa include blisters, bullas, pustules, vesicles, papules, plaques, and hematomas. Shallow lesions are significant because they may be contagious, are painful, and can prevent the patient from obtaining proper nutrition. Blisters are thin-walled, fluid-filled sacs resulting from friction or viral diseases. Fluid accumulation occurs when blood vessels leak following trauma. Vesicles, bullas, and pustules are all variations of blisters. Vesicles are small blisters filled with fluid or gas and usually come from herpes or Varicella. Bullae are larger, with diameters larger than 0.5 inch. Pustules are infected blisters containing dead white cells and bacteria as pus. Hematomas are reddish lesions containing a semi-solid mass of blood from a ruptured blood vessel; hematomas commonly appear after application of oral anesthetic. A plaque is any elevated (or level) lesion in the oral mucosa.

Deep lesions that appear underneath the surface of the oral mucosa include abscesses, cysts, ulcers and erosions. Abscesses are pus-filled cavities resulting from bacterial infection and inflammation; in the oral cavity. Most abscesses appear near the apex of the tooth or in the periodontal area. They require high dose antibiotic treatment (usually penicillin) to avoid bone loss, septicemia, and possible heart, kidney, and brain infection. Cysts are thick-walled cavities that contain fluid or a semi-solid, fluid mixture. Cyst formation usually occurs from duct blockage, but can result from other diseases. Ulcers occur when mucous membranes are damaged. Ulcers are reddened, painful, open sores. Erosions are indentations left after trauma; they have red and tender borders.

The types of oral lesions observable on the surface flats of the oral mucosa include macules, ecchymosis, patches, petechiae, purpura, granulomas, neoplasms and nodules. The latter three may also present above the surface of the oral mucosa.

Macules are spots and patches are irregular areas that differ in texture and/or color from their surroundings. An example is white thrush, yeast that colonizes patients with depressed immune systems. Ecchymosis is bruised tissue. Pinpoint hemorrhaging is petechiae. Purpura is small red or purple spots, which includes tiny petechiae, and larger areas of discoloration up to an inch in diameter, such as ecchymosis. Neoplasms are tumorous growths, either benign (noncancerous) or malignant (cancerous). A granuloma is one type of neoplasm, in which chronic inflammation produces an area of granulation tissue. Nodules are small protuberances of either hard or soft tissue. The dentist refers the patient with a neoplasm to an M.D. for investigation.

Oral lesions are caused by dental procedures, radiation injury, or trauma, which can be self-induced. Incorrect use of dental instruments can tear or bruise the oral mucosa. Incorrect removal of cotton rolls, used to dry tissue, can induce ulcers in the gums. Improperly fitted or worn dentures can cause ulcers. Eventually, folds of extra tissue (hyperplasia) form. The palate develops red, swollen lumps. Particles of silver amalgam, used to fill caries, can catch in tissue and discolor it blue or gray, but an amalgam tattoo poses no health issue. Excess radiation therapy for head and neck cancer damages the teeth roots or ulcerates the target area. Self-induced traumas to the oral cavity include biting the inside of the cheek or contact with a dull object, such as mouth jewelry in piercings. Ask your patient to remove mouth jewelry before imaging.

Use of tobacco is the main chemical cause of oral lesions. Nicotine stomatitis is common in pipe smokers and, to a lesser extent, cigarette smokers. Mouth areas repeatedly exposed to the heat and chemicals in tobacco initially redden from irritation. Later, they develop white and red, thick bumps containing keratin protein (hyperkeratinized). The patient's salivary gland openings may also become inflamed. Another type of tobacco-related lesion can occur with use of snuff or chewing tobacco. The lesion occurs generally in the lower front mouth, between lips and teeth, and is similar to nicotine stomatitis. Irritations from smoking marijuana can look very similar to tobacco use, although marijuana lesions usually occur inside both lips.

Hairy tongue (lingua villosa) is lengthened, darkened tongue papillae. A thick coating covers the tongue's middle dorsum, especially near the throat. It may be black brown, green, white, or pink. Papillae wave if you shoot a blast of compressed air at them. Causes include: Broad spectrum antibiotics; tobacco; intravenous drugs; coffee; tea; breath mints; candies; hydrogen peroxide rinses; low fiber diet; poor oral hygiene; and HIV. Your patient has halitosis (bad breath) because long papillae trap food. Your patient complains of gagging or tickling when he/she swallows. Instruct your patient to brush his/her tongue and eliminate the agents to cure hairy tongue.

The seizure medication phenytoin (Dilantin), orthodontic braces, or plaque can cause gingival hyperplasia. Connective tissue from the gum extends over the teeth, affecting eating and appearance. If the irritant (e.g., an essential drug) cannot be removed, surgical removal is an option.

Patients who put acetylsalicylic acid (ASA) over aching roots develop Aspirin burn, in which coarse, white lesions form.

About 1 in 20 pregnant women develops pregnancy gingivitis, in which the gum tissues become inflated and inflamed. Occasionally, tumors develop. Pregnancy gingivitis should subside when hormone levels return to normal.

Another type of lesion often found in pregnant women is pyogenic granuloma. However, it can also affect nonpregnant women and men. Pyogenic granuloma is a rapidly growing, reddened, vascular mass of granulation tissue. It results from a combination of hormonal changes and local irritation.

Gingival swelling can also occur during the hormonal changes associated with puberty, primarily in girls. Once hormonal balance is restored, the gingival enlargement should subside.

Lumpy Jaw and Syphilis

Lumpy jaw is an abscess caused by a bacterial infection, called actinomycosis. The usual culprit is the anaerobic bacterium Actinomyces israelii. Actinomyces species are commensal mouth and throat flora that neither hurt nor help their host. However, after surgery or trauma, Actinomyces can become a pathogen that causes swollen, reddish-purple lumps, pus-draining skin sores with yellow "sulfur" granules, fever, and weight loss. Lumpy jaw produces little or no pain. The dental assistant swabs the sore for culture and sensitivity testing. The doctor may lance the lump. The patient needs antibiotics for several months up to one year to clear actinomycosis. Left untreated, it infects the lungs and causes sores on the chest wall.

Syphilis is a venereal disease transmitted by sexual or mother-to-fetus contact with Treponema pallidum spirochetes. Syphilis has three stages:
Lip chancres (firm, raised lesions that develop ulcers and crusting)
Infectious patches or papules
Localized gummas or tumors
Children of syphilitic mothers have tooth enamel hypoplasia, or Hutchinson's incisor's (ragged incisal edges), or mulberry molars.

Oral Viruses and Fungi

The herpes family causes most oral viral infections:

- Herpes simplex type I is primarily a mouth ulcer but can be transmitted by oral sex. Herpes simplex type I is contracted by physical contact in childhood. Eruptions occur throughout life. Burning vesicles are followed by crusted cold sores on the lips or in the mouth. Wear PPE when treating herpetic patients. You can develop ulcers on your hands and eyes, if infected.

- Herpes simplex type II, the genital variety, can appear in the mouth.
- Herpes zoster is shingles and usually affects the elderly. It is a reactivation of childhood Varicella (chickenpox). Herpes zoster lesions are usually one-sided along the course of a nerve, very painful, and long lasting.

Candidiasis (thrush) is a thick, white monilia yeast infection coating the mucous membranes of breastfeeding children and immunosuppressed patients. Gently scrape the plaque. Apply topical antifungals. AIDS patients may have chronic Herpes simplex, Herpes zoster, and thrush infections, causing weight loss.

Aphthous Ulcers

Aphthous ulcers are canker sores, painful oral ulcerations of unknown origin. Aphthous ulcers have lesions with yellow centers encircled by red halos. The yellow center is actually necrosis of epithelial cells. Aphthous ulcers do not appear to be contagious. Causative agents have not been positively identified. However, Streptococci are often been found in the ulcers. Other factors that promote aphthous ulcer formation are stress, hormonal changes, and food allergies. Aphthous ulcers recur periodically when the patient experiences one of these triggers. Aphthous ulcers typically persist for 10 to 14 days. Sooth aphthous ulcers with topical anesthetics, e.g., Anbesol. Postpone oral procedures during exacerbations, as aphthous ulcers are very painful.

Congenital Conditions

Congenital conditions are genetically inherited states. Nine common congenital abnormalities found in the oral cavity include:

- Cleft lip (hare lip) or cleft palate
- Unusually large teeth (macrodontia)
- Unusually small teeth (microdontia) often associated with Down syndrome or congenital heart disease. Amelogenesis imperfecta and dentinogenesis imperfect, hereditary conditions thinning the enamel, discoloring it (amelogenesis), or making it opalescent (dentinogenesis) and prone to caries and enamel wear
- Congenitally missing teeth (anodontia)
- Extra teeth (supernumerary), present at birth and quickly shed
- Fusion of two or more teeth
- Ankylosis, the fusion of a tooth, cementum, or dentin to the alveolar bone
- Gemination, in which a tooth bud cannot fully divide
- Twinning, the development of two distinct teeth from one tooth bud

Cleft Lip and Cleft Palate

Both cleft lip and cleft palate are developmental failures of tissues in the oral cavity to fuse properly. Cleft lip occurs when maxillary processes in the head do not fuse with the medial nasal process, resulting in a notching or more pronounced indentation from the lip to nostril. It can be unilateral (on one side) or bilateral (on both sides). Cleft palate occurs when the palatal shelves do not fuse with the primary palate or each other. It can be found alone or in combination with cleft lip. There are different types of cleft palate, depending on the fusion failure. The least severe is cleft uvula, in which only the uvular flap at the back of the soft palate fails to fuse. More serious variations include: Bilateral cleft of the secondary palate; bilateral cleft lip, alveolar process, and primary palate; bilateral cleft of the lip, alveolar process and both primary and secondary palates; unilateral cleft lip, primary palate, and alveolar process. The infant requires maxillofacial surgery.

Oral Tori and Exostosis

Oral tori are benign, boney extensions into the oral cavity covered with fine layers of tissue. Extensions developing from the maxillary hard palate are called torus palatinus. They occur in about 20% of adults and are usually near the midline. Torus mandibularis, outgrowths in canine or premolar areas of the mandible, are less common but more bothersome, because food fragments imbed there. Both oral tori can cause tenderness during oral radiography. They should be surgically excised if dental appliances are necessary. Exostosis is the swelling or nodular outgrowth of the lamella bone on the facial side of the maxillary or mandibular palates. It is very similar to oral tori.

Developmental Abnormalities

One of the most common developmental abnormalities involving the tongue is fissured tongue, in which the tongue surface is deeply grooved and sometimes asymmetrical (unevenly shaped). A bifid tongue occurs when the sides of the front of the tongue do not fuse fully, and a tip of muscle is exposed at the end of the tongue. Usually, both of these conditions are left untreated. Ankyloglossia is the connection of the lingual frenulum close to the tip of the tongue, impeding its movement, and preventing the speaker from making certain sounds clearly. It can be corrected with a simple surgical procedure that cuts the frenulum. The vast majority of affected patients also have an abnormality called Fordyce's spots or granules, sebaceous oil glands close to surface epithelia in the oral mucosa.

Improper Diet

The most common oral conditions caused by improper diet are angular cheilitis and glossitis. Angular cheilitis is due to a shortage of Vitamin B complex. It presents as a lesion of both the mucous membranes and skin near the corner of the mouth, thus changing the vertical dimension of the face. Saliva accumulates at the corners and microorganisms proliferate there, particularly opportunistic infections like Candida albicans. The deficiency must be corrected and antifungal drugs are prescribed. Angular cheilitis can also develop if the person often licks the corners of his/her mouth, or drops vertical length in his/her face. Vitamin B complex deficiency is probably also the cause of glossitis or bald tongue, in which the tongue is inflamed and filiform papillae are lacking.

Oral Cancer

Suspect oral cancer (malignancy) if your patient displays any of the following warning signals:

- A sore in the oral cavity that does not resolve within about a month

- Protracted mouth dryness

- Lumps or areas of swelling in the region, including lips, oral cavity, or neck

- White or coarse lesions on the lips or in the oral cavity

- Numbness

- Tenderness

- Burning sensations in or anywhere near the oral cavity

- Unexplained, recurrent bleeding in one part of the mouth

- Difficulty speaking

- Difficulty chewing or swallowing (dysphagia)

Report your findings to the dentist immediately. The dentist must refer the patient to an M.D. for follow-up.

Oral Tumors

Oral tumors are called neoplasms. Benign tumors are not cancerous, but can still cause pain, deformity, and loss of normal use. Some benign tumors have the potential for malignancy:

- Squamous papillomae are benign tumors that develop after human papilloma virus (HPV) infections, usually types 6 and 11. Projections of squamous epithelial tissue can be surgically removed.
- Fibromas are benign areas of hyperplasia; they present as pink, even, dome-shaped lesions, generally on the buccal surface.
- Lichen planus looks like a flattened, deep reed or violet bump. Often, lichen planus is found on the patient's leg or ankle. In the mouth, the buccal mucosa is usually involved, and lines know as Wickham's striae may be seen. The patient usually has soreness while eating. The dentist usually prescribes topical steroids. Its malignant potential is unclear.

Squamous cell and basal cell carcinomas are malignant tumors. Squamous epithelial cell carcinoma is the predominant oral cancer. It metastasizes (spreads through the lymph nodes) quickly. Predisposing factors include tobacco use, alcohol use, and exposure to sunlight. Squamous cell carcinomas initially look like white plaques that later ulcerate. Basal cell carcinoma is the chief form of skin cancer, again caused primarily by sunlight exposure. Fortunately, basal cell carcinoma rarely metastasizes and lesions can be surgically removed. Red patches in the oral cavity that are not due to inflammation are erythroplakia. Red patches are usually found on the floor of the mouth, the soft palate, or retro molar pad. They are associated with chronic tobacco or alcohol use, and they are almost without exception malignant or premalignant. Early erythroplakia is treated surgically. Late stage erythroplakia receives radiation and chemotherapy. Leukoplakia is unidentifiable white, tough, hyperkeratinized patches in the mucosa that cannot be wiped off, and are potentially malignant.

Human immunodeficiency virus (HIV) suppresses the immune response of acquired immunodeficiency syndrome (AIDS) patients, so they are susceptible to opportunistic infections unusual for adults in their prime. For example, oral thrush (Candida albicans) usually affects nursing babies, and Kaposi's sarcoma usually affects elderly Mediterranean men. HIV infection is transmissible by blood and is incurable, so wear PPE. Good dental hygiene is imperative for AIDS patients because they are especially vulnerable to periodontal lesions due to bacterial and fungal infections. Chemotherapy or long-term antibiotic use trigger Candida in the oral mucosa. Look for thick, white lines superimposed over red, inflamed areas, particularly on the tongue or cheeks. Give antifungals, like Nystatin. HIV-positive patients often have hairy leukoplakia or white patterns near the edges of the tongue. The vascular malignancy Kaposi's sarcoma presents as scattered bluish-purple lesions on the palate, nose, and arms that bleed. Low-dose radiation and/or chemotherapy are indicated.

Miscellaneous Disorders

One of the most common miscellaneous disorders is geographic tongue, in which smooth red patches bounded by yellow or white edges cover the back and sides of the tongue and filiform papillae (hairy extensions) are missing. Geographic tongue does not hurt and requires no intervention.

Acute necrotizing ulcerative gingivitis (ANUG) often occurs in teenagers and young adults and is infectious. ANUG is characterized by oral cavity pain, infection, bleeding, and a foul odor. Clean and débride the affected area. Give antibiotics and hot water rinses.

A mucocele is a bump inside the upper lip from a salivary duct closed by trauma, such as lip biting. The dentist may lance the salivary gland to drain accumulated fluid.

Varix is weakened and distended blood vessels in the mouth.

Bell's palsy causes drooping features because of temporary paralysis of facial muscles on one side.

Anorexia nervosa is an eating disorder characterized by unrealistic fears of consuming food and weight loss of at least 15%. Bulimia is an eating disorder distinguished by uncontrollable binge eating followed by self-induced vomiting. Eating disorder patients can die from electrolyte imbalance and heart attack. The appearance of the oral cavity changes due to vomiting accompanying bulimia: The lingual surfaces of the front teeth lose calcium; enamel wears away; occlusal faces of back teeth also erode. If the patient had restorative work, the fillings fail. Eating disordered patients tend to have many caries and enlarged parotid glands. Good oral hygiene is imperative, particularly after vomiting. Recommend toothpaste for sensitive teeth to eating disordered patients.

Periodontal Diseases

Periodontal diseases involve the periodontium, the tissue that surrounds and holds up the teeth. Periodontal diseases can lead to tooth loss through lack of support. Most periodontal disease starts as inflammation resulting from the buildup of plaque, bacterial colonies sticking to teeth or areas of the gingivae. Mineralized plaque on teeth is called dental calculus. Caries can develop from plaque when sugars are converted into acids by the bacteria. Periodontal disease can also result from hormonal disturbances or other oral problems. Risk factors include: Diabetes; poor oral hygiene; osteoporosis; stress; certain medications; HIV/AIDS; irritation from dental appliances; and malocclusion. One type of periodontal disease involves the gums (gingivae); the presence of inflamed and bleeding gums is gingivitis. If the bacterial infection spreads to the underlying supporting alveolar bone, periodontitis results.

Periodontitis

In addition to the gingiva and alveolar bone, other structures in the periodontium may be involved in periodontitis. These include the epithelial attachment, the periodontal ligaments in contact with the root and alveolar bone, and the cementum or bony tissue covering the roots. Periodontal disease classification is related to:
- Involvement of all of these structures
- How aggressive the disease is
- Whether or not necrosis has occurred
- The size of the sulcus or space dividing the tooth and free gingiva

Class I or chronic periodontitis is characterized inflammation of the area, destruction of the periodontal ligament, bone damage and tooth mobility. Class I is subdivided into slight, moderate, and severe categories, based on depth of pockets of detachment, degree of bone loss, tooth mobility, and for molars furcation involvement. Class II or aggressive periodontitis is early-onset and rapidly progressing destruction of tissue and clinical signs of inflammation. It can occur as local prepubertal periodontitis, occurring between the eruption of primary teeth and puberty, or as juvenile periodontitis (either localized or systemic). Class III or necrotizing periodontal disease is ulcerative tissue death.

Excessive dental plaque leads to periodontal disease. Indicate plaque on the chart by a squiggly line above the tooth. Indicate periodontal pockets with an arrow and number indicating depths. A full periodontal chart enumerates the periodontal pocket depth for each tooth on both the facial and lingual sides. The dentist or hygienist "walks" the probe around the tooth and takes six distinct sulcal measurements (mesio-buccal, midbuccal, distobuccal, distolingual, mid-lingual, and mesio-lingual). Classify tooth mobility as normal (0), slight (1), moderate (2) or severe (3). Note areas of exudate or pus. Show gingival recession by drawing a dotted or colored line along the gum line, to illustrate root exposure. Note furcation involvement for the molars only.

Periodontal Examination

A periodontal examination consists of the history, radiographs, examination, measurements, charting, and assessment and scaling by the dentist. Good radiographs can show evidence of periodontal disease. Examination of the teeth includes assessment of tooth mobility with two instruments, inspection of the gingivae and supporting structures, and looking for and probing periodontal pockets. Periodontal probes standardized in millimeters are used to measure depths of six surfaces, the facial, lingual, distofacial, distolingual, semiofficial and mesiolingual. The dental assistant logs the deepest pockets on the periodontal chart, along with pocket depths, furcations, mobility, exudates, and gingival recession. The dentist uses explorers to find calculus and assess the root, straight or curved scalers to get rid of supragingival calculus, and less blunt curettes to remove subgingival calculus.

Normal Occlusion

Occlusion is the relationship between upper and lower teeth when the mouth is closed. In normal occlusion, teeth in both dental arches are in maximum contact, without rotation or nonstandard spacing. The front teeth in the maxillary arch overlap the incisal edge of those in the mandible slightly, by about 2 millimeters. The maxillary posterior teeth are positioned one cusp further back than the mandibular posterior ones. Lastly, the mesial buccal cusp of the first permanent molar in the upper arch is in contact with the buccal groove of the first molar in the mandible. Normal occlusion should give a mesognathic facial profile, a straight line between jaws with only a slight projection of the mandible, relative to the upper part of the face.

Malocclusion

Malocclusion is any divergence from normal occlusion. Angle's classifications are used most often to describe three basic types of malocclusion:

Neutroclusion (Class I), in which occlusion is essentially normal, except that individual or groups of teeth are out of position and the facial profile is still mesognathic.

Distoclusion (Class II), in which the buccal groove of the mandibular first permanent molar is behind the mesiobuccal cusp of the corresponding maxillary molar.

Distoclusion can be Division 1 or 2, due to either outward protrusion of the maxillary teeth or backward sloping of the mandibular teeth. Both produce a retrognathic facial profile, where one or both jaws are recessed.

Mesioclusion (Class III), in which the buccal groove of the mandibular first permanent molar is mesial to the mesiobuccal cusp of the corresponding maxillary molar. The facial profile is prognathic, meaning the jaws project beyond the upper part of the face.

Malocclusion is caused by one of three factors:

1. Inherited genetic factors can contribute to formation of extra or supernumerary teeth, missing teeth, atypical relationships between the jaws, or between teeth and the jaw, and deviations such as cleft palate.
2. Exposure to systemic diseases or nutritional deficiencies during the formative years can interrupt the normal developmental pattern of dentition.
3. Particular habits or localized trauma can produce malocclusion. These

include mouth breathing, thumb or tongue sucking, thrusting of the tongue, nail biting, and bruxism. Bruxism is the unconscious grinding of teeth during sleep or stressful situations.

Malpositions

Individual teeth can exhibit the following variations and contribute to malocclusion:
- Teeth that are mesial, distal, or lingual to their normal position are examples of mesioversion, distoversion and linguoversion, respectively.
- Torsoversion is the rotation or turning of a tooth from the expected position.
- Buccoversion or labioversion is the inclination of a tooth toward the cheek or lip. If the crown of an individual tooth is outside the normal line of occlusion, it exhibits either supraversion (above) or infraversion (below).
- Finally, a tooth may appear in the wrong position or order of the dental arch, a variation called transversion or transposition.

Overbite and overjet are two types of malpositions between groups of teeth that result in malocclusion. Both are teeth overlaps. An overbite is a greater than normal vertical overlap between anterior maxillary and mandibular teeth. An overbite means the upper incisors extend over more than one-third of the front teeth in the mandible. An overjet is horizontal overlap, with an unusually large horizontal distance between the outer surface of the anterior mandibular teeth and the inner face of the maxillary anterior teeth. A person can also have an underjet, where the front teeth in the mandible project significantly in front of the maxillary anterior teeth.

A cross-bite is an atypical relationship between single teeth or groups of teeth in one dental arch, relative to the other. With a cross-bite involving anterior teeth, the incisors in the maxilla are lingual to the opposing ones in the mandible. Posterior cross-bite presents similarly, with maxillary back teeth closer to the tongue than the mandibular teeth, the opposite of that expected with a normal bite. There can also be an:
- Edge-edge bite, in which the incisal surfaces of teeth in both arches converge
- End-to-end bite between posterior teeth whose cusps meet
- Open bite, in which there is a lack of occlusion between the mandibular and maxillary teeth.

Facial Landmarks

The dentist notes abnormalities of these landmarks of the face and oral cavity during examination:
The first facial landmark is the outside edge or ala of the nose
Extending from the nose to the corner of the mouth is the naso-labial groove
The philtrum is the hollow between the bottom of the nose and the center of the upper lip
Lips have four landmarks: (1) the vermillion zone, the entire reddish part of the lips, (2) the vermillion border surrounding it, (3) the tubercle of the lip, the slight protrusion in the center of the upper lip, and (4) the labial commissures, the corners of the mouth. The lip vermillion zone is highly vascularized, which makes it pink or red in a healthy person, and blue in a cold, hypoxic, or dead person.
The final facial landmark is the labio-mental groove, a horizontal depression in the middle between the lip and chin

Oral Cavity Landmarks

The oral cavity has a vestibule or mucobuccal fold, the pouch where the soft cheek and gums meet. Its continuous border is the

vestibule fornix. There mucosa (moist linings) in the oral cavity are:
(1) the labial mucosa on the inside of the lips
(2) the buccal mucosa on the interior of the cheeks
(3) the looser, redder alveolar mucosa encasing the alveolar bone, shoring up the teeth.

On the labial mucosa, near the corners of the mouth, are Fordyce's spots, minute yellow glands. The buccal mucosa has two characteristic features: An elevated white line where teeth meet, called the linea alba, and a piece of skin across from the maxillary second molar, known as the parotid papilla. Another landmark is the gingiva, which are pink, fibrous gum tissue surrounding teeth. The oral cavity has two types of frena (restraining folds of tissue): The labial frena (the major ones between the central incisors in either jaw) and the buccal frena. Frenulum and frenum are both correct singulars of frena.

The palate is the roof of the mouth, interior to the maxillary teeth. The front or hard palate is comprised of a bony plate, enveloped with pink keratinized tissue, and the back or soft palate, made of muscle.

Hard Palate Landmarks	Soft Palate Landmarks
Incisive papilla (an elevated area behind the top central incisors), ridges that run either down the center toward the back	Uvula, an outcrop of tissue at the entrance to the throat
A single palatine raphe, running horizontally across the hard palate posterior to the incisive papilla, the palatine rugae	Anterior tonsillar pillars that arch toward the tongue, and posterior tonsillar pillars extending behind the soft palate into the oropharynx
Torus palatinus, a bony protuberance in the center of the palate	Palatine tonsils located between the posterior pillars at the rear of the oral cavity in the fauces, the entrance to the pharynx.

The dorsal (top) side of the tongue has several types of papilla or projections in its anterior two-thirds, bearing the taste buds. The dorsal tongue has a groove, called the median sulcus, dividing the front portion in half, and another groove in the back, called the sulcus terminalis. Large circumvallated papillae are located in front of the sulcus terminalis. Hair-like protrusions, called filiform papillae, appear further forward. Redder, fungiform papillae appear near the front of the tongue. Tissue creases on the sides of the tongue are foliate papillae. The ventral (underside) of the tongue has a central line of tissue, termed the lingual frenum, which continues into the floor of the mouth. There are lingual veins on its sides, and tissue creases, called fimbriated folds. At the point of attachment where the lingual frenum meets the floor of the mouth, there are tissue folds called sublingual caruncles. Sublingual folds branch from the caruncles.

There is a sublingual sulcus close to the dental arch.

Salivary glands secrete saliva, a digestive fluid, into the oral cavity. Saliva moistens food and tissues in the oral space, facilitates chewing and ingestion, aids digestion of starches, and normalizes water balance. Saliva is a transparent liquid, normally of slightly alkaline pH. Saliva contains water, mucin protein, organic salts, and ptyalin enzyme. Saliva is secreted from three pairs of salivary glands and their adjoining ducts, which drain the saliva into the mouth. The parotid glands are located ahead of the ear; their parotid or Stensen's ducts empty into the area around the maxillary second molars. The submandibular glands are located in the rear of the mandible; their Warton's ducts drain into the sublingual caruncles. The sublingual glands are positioned on the floor of the mouth and can empty either right into the mouth via the ducts of Rivinus, or indirectly via the ducts of Bartholin into the sublingual caruncles.

Maxilla

The maxilla (upper jaw) is the biggest facial bone, extending from the eye sockets and nasal cavities to form the roof of the oral cavity. The maxilla has two segments of bone, held together in the middle by the median suture. The maxilla develops from four bony outgrowths or processes: Frontal, zygomatic, alveolar, and palatine. The infraorbital foramen open beneath the eye sockets. Sizeable maxillary sinuses open near the roots of the top molars, and there is a rounded area in the back, called the maxillary tuberosity. The palatine bones fuse at the midline along the palatine suture. The nasopalatine nerve connects to the palatine bones near the front at the incisive foramen. There is a horizontally located transverse palatine suture near the back of the hard palate. Posterior to it on each side are three other openings, one greater palatine foramen, and two more diminutive, lesser palatine foramen.

Mandible

The only facial bone that can move is the mandible (lower jaw). It curves in front in the horizontal plane (following the dental arch), with vertical wings at the back, called rami. The rami are capped by two projections, the condyloid process in the back (which connects to the temporal bone to form the temporomandibular joint) and the sharper coronoid process, anterior to it. From the ramus area going forward, are the mandibular and mental foramen on the outside, and the lingual foramen on the tongue side. The latter has characteristic ridges. The front of the mandible is distinguished by a depression in its center, where the symphysis bones meet. The apex of the chin is the mental protuberance.

Cranial Bones

Cranial bones enclose and protect the brain, and produce some red blood cells. There are two temporal bones at the lower sides and base of the skull and one frontal bone in the forehead. There are two parietal bones on the top and upper sides of the head. The occipital bone lies at the rear and base of the skull. The sphenoid bone is in front of the temporal area. The ethmoid bones create part of the nose, eye sockets, and floor of the cranium. Various processes and sinuses make the cranium light. There are eight types of facial bones: A set of nasal bones constituting the bridge of the nose; one vomer bone inside, forming part of the nasal septum that separates the two nasal cavities; inferior nasal conchae inside the cavity that warm and filter air; two lacrimal bones that are part of the orbit of the eye; zygomatic bones create the cheeks and are also part of the maxilla or upper jaw; two maxilla; the palatine bones; and the mandible.

Temporomandibular Joint

The temporomandibular joint (TMJ) is a junction formed by the glenoid fossa, and articular eminence of the temporal bone, and the condyloid process of the mandible. The temporal bones on either side of the face are cranial bones. The TMJ is immersed in synovial fluid, and its bones are enclosed by cartilage and supported by ligaments. The condyloid process or condyle is padded with fibrous connective tissue, called the articular disc or meniscus. When the mouth is closed, the meniscus is in close contact with the glenoid fossa of the temporal bone and the articular eminence further forward. The meniscus and glenoid are separated by cavities bathed in synovial fluid. As the mouth opens, a hinge motion develops, as the condyles and discs move forward. Then the condyles and discs move further forward, as the mouth opens more in a forward gliding joint movement. If the meniscus gets trapped or dislocated, TMJ disease manifests as a clicking noise and jaw pain.

TMJ (temporomandibular joint) dysfunction is lack of coordination in the structures associated with the TMJ. It can present as: Pain near the ear, often extending into the face; soreness in the chewing muscles; popping or clicking noises when opening or closing the mouth; crepitus (grating); tinnitus (ringing in the ears); headache or neck pain; inability to adequately open the mouth (trismus) or move the lower jaw. Diagnosis of TMJ dysfunction or disease is based on a combination of medical and dental history, physical examination, evaluation by tomographic radiography or magnetic resonance imaging, and casts of the teeth to replicate the movements of the jaws. In particular, ask your patient about grinding or clamping the teeth, bite issues, injuries, diseases, and stress when you take the history. The clinician examines the area by palpation, takes note of characteristic sounds while the jaw is opened and closed, and quantifies how wide the patient can open his/her mouth.

Some treatment options for TMJ dysfunction are relatively minor, such as: Stress management; rotating heat and cold application; resting the jaw; and NSAID pain relievers, muscle relaxants, antibiotics, mood enhancers, and anti-anxiety drugs. Physiotherapy and massage are often helpful. If minor treatments do not alleviate pain, the dentist progresses to steroid injections into the intra-articular area. The dentist may apply occlusal splints to alleviate spasms or pressure. Often, TMJ disorders are treatable with orthodontia and other restoration. For extreme cases that do not respond to conventional treatments, several types of surgery can be attempted by a maxillofacial surgeon. TMJ surgeries include arthroscopic removal of adhesions, coupled with insertion of anti-inflammatory agents, and open joint surgery, in which the joints are actually reconstructed.

Chairside Dental Procedures

Treatment Room Equipment

A comfortable, supportive dental chair with arm supports and an adjustable headrest and controls. The chair must accommodate upright, supine and sub supine positions. Ergonomic chairs or stools for both operator and assistant. The operator's (dentist's) chair should have 5 castors, an adjustable seat and back, and a broad base. The assistant needs a chair with a foot bar for support.
Track-mounted, iridescent operating light to illuminate the oral cavity
An air-water syringe to provide streams of water and/or air
An oral evacuation system that includes a saliva ejector and a high velocity evacuation (HVE) device
A curing light, an electronically-controlled blue light-emitting wand that polymerizes resins and composites
Various handpieces operated by a foot-controlled rheostat or resistor attached to the dental unit
If restorations are performed, an amalgamator to make the materials

Proper Seated Positions

The dental operator (dentist, hygienist, or nurse) sits with a straight back, feet planted on the floor, and knees slightly below hip level. Adjust the chair height level so the patient's mouth is level with the operator's elbows. The operator should be relaxed, with eyes directed downward toward the patient.

The assistant sits 4 to 5 inches higher than the operator to permit greater visibility and access. Sit up straight, with the abdominal bar or chair back in a supportive position. Place your feet on the base platform, not the floor. Keep your hips and thighs parallel to the floor, level with the patient's shoulders.

Dental operators experience shoulder, neck and back pain. Shoulder and neck pain is due to extended strain or flexion. Combined neck and back pain is due to prolonged extension or lifting of the arm. Low back pain is due to prolonged twisting. Carpal tunnel syndrome is a repetitive strain injury from prolonged wrist flexion and extension, as when keyboarding.

Operating Zones

Team or four-handed dentistry requires four distinct zones in the treatment area:
1. A static zone right behind the patient, where the dental unit and a moveable cabinet are located.
2. The operator's zone is the largest segment, to the left or right of the static zone, where the operator (dentist/hygienist/nurse) sits and moves around. Placement depends on whether the dentist is right-handed or left-handed.
3. The assistant's zone is directly opposite the operator with the instrument cart and dental materials.
4. A transfer zone next to the assistant is over the patient's chest, where assistant and operator exchange dental materials and instruments.

These four operating zones are often described in terms of a clock face with 12 divisions: The static zone occupies 2 portions; the operator occupies 5 portions; and the combined assistant and transfer zones making up the remainder (5 portions).

Instrument Transfer Techniques

The assistant should transfer instruments within the transfer zone over the patient's chest. Both operator and assistant wear gloves. Transfer instruments with minimal motion. Keep the working end pointed toward the tooth being repaired. Keep the handle available for the dentist to grasp. In the single-handed transfer technique, the clinical assistant picks up the instrument from the tray, using the thumb and first two fingers of the left hand. The assistant holds the handle end or the side not required and places it into the transfer zone, near the implement in use. Exchange the instruments by using the last two fingers of the left hand for retrieval of the used one. Fold the used instrument into your palm. Simultaneously, put the new tool into the operator's fingers. Return the used instrument to its correct position in the setup tray. In the two-handed technique, grip the new instrument similarly in your right hand. Recover the used implement with your left hand and return it to the tray by releasing the palm grasp. Give the new instrument to the dentist with proper orientation of the working end.

The operator uses the mouth mirror and explorer for examination at the beginning of the procedure. These are transferred from the assistant to dentist at the same time, using the two-handed technique. Most instruments are gripped by the dentist in a pen, palm, or palm-and-thumb grasp. The assistant holds pliers and forceps over their hinges and puts the handles directly into the dentist's palm or over his/her fingers. To transfer using cotton pliers, squeeze the beaks together to avoid dropping the cotton. Transfer dental materials much closer to the chin than instruments. The dental assistant can either give amalgam to the dentist or, if allowed by state law, directly insert it into the tooth. Transfer impression materials and cements delivered via syringes directly to the dentist, with the tip facing the arch where he/she is working. Convey cements and liners on mixing slabs, along with the applicator device. The assistant uses his/her right hand to hold the slab. The left hand wipes off any excess with gauze.

Mouth Rinsing Methods

The dental assistant is responsible for both mouth rinsing and oral evacuation during dental procedures. Use either a saliva ejector or a more powerful high-volume oral evacuator (HVE). Perform limited-area rinsing often during pauses in the procedure to eliminate debris. Perform a complete mouth rinse at the end of the procedure. Grip the air-water syringe in your left hand and the saliva or HVE in your right hand. For a limited rinse, point the tip toward the desired area and direct air and water to the site. Suction out fluid and debris. Dry the site by compressing the air button. Place the patient facing you during the final full-mouth rinse. Direct the HVE or saliva ejector tip into left part of the oral cavity (without touching tissues). Direct the air-water syringe first from right to left, along the maxillary arch, and then right to left along the mandibular arch. Place the suction tip in the back of the mouth to remove the fluid and extracted debris.

Oral Evacuation Methods

Moisture control and maintenance of a clinical field are paramount during dental procedures. A saliva ejector is a small flexible tube attached to a bulb, used for oral evacuation of minute quantities of saliva or water. A high-volume oral evacuator (HVE) is needed for large quantities of saliva and water, or for blood, pus, and vomitus. The HVE is essentially a vacuum with a sterile tip attached. Tips can be made of plastic or stainless steel. Tips are either straight or slightly angled, and the working end slants. Hold the evacuator with either a pen or thumb-to-nose grasp in the same hand as the dentist uses. Use your other hand to operate the air-water syringe or for instrument transfer. The patient's tongue and cheek must be isolated from the evacuation site

- 26 -

with the HVE tip or the mouth mirror. There are several techniques for HVE tip placement, including on the lingual or buccal surfaces, slightly behind the prepped area, or on the opposite side of the tooth.

High-Volume Evacuator

When you use an HVE (high-volume oral evacuator) in posterior areas, position the beveled edge of the tip as near to the tooth being prepared as possible, and parallel to either the buccal or lingual surface. The upper edge of the tip should reach a bit beyond the occlusal surface. Place a cotton roll under the tip for comfort when mandibular areas are being controlled. For anterior or front teeth, position the HVE tip parallel to the opposite surface and somewhat beyond the incisal edge of the tooth being prepared. Lingual and facial preparations require vacuum extraction from the facial and lingual sides, respectively.

Cotton Rolls

Cotton rolls isolate and control moisture in a working area during an oral procedure. For maxillary placement, the patient faces the assistant with his/her chin elevated. The assistant uses cotton pliers to grasp and convey the cotton roll to the mucobuccal fold nearest the working area of the patient's mouth. For mandibular placement, the patient faces the assistant with his/her chin lowered. The assistant picks up the cotton roll with the cotton pliers and transfers the roll to the corresponding mucobuccal fold. Place a second cotton roll on the floor of the mouth, between the operational field and the tongue. Ask the patient to raise his/her tongue to facilitate placement. Bend cotton rolls used in anterior regions before positioning. Take rolls out before the final full-mouth rinse, using cotton pliers. Very dry rolls can stick to the oral mucosa causing tissue damage. If a roll sticks, moisten it with water from the air-water syringe before removal.

Dry Angles

Dry angles are triangular-shaped, absorbent pads that may be used during oral procedures in the back areas of either dental arch. Position the angles on top of the Stensen's duct, on the inside of the cheek, near the maxillary second molar. One type of salivary gland, the parotid gland, leads to the Stensen's duct. Therefore, the main purpose of dry angles is to obstruct the saliva flow into the area. The pads also preserve the oral tissues. Replace dry angles that become saturated with saliva. Moisten them further with the air-water syringe before removal.

Dental Dams

Dental dams are commercially-available barriers used to isolate areas during oral procedures. The dam improves access for the dentist and assistant because it retracts the lips, tongue and gums. It also enhances visibility of the area by providing color contrast. Dams come in latex or latex-free materials in various sizes, colors and thicknesses. Dams are divided into sixths, with holes punched for placement in the upper or lower middle portion for maxillary or mandibular treatments, respectively. Employ dental dams for involved procedures requiring local anesthesia. The patient is less likely to accidentally inhale or swallow materials when a dental dam is used. A dental dam provides infection and moisture control. It inhibits contact with debris and dental materials. In some states, the dental assistant may legally place the dental dam.

The dental dam is held in a three-sided, plastic or metal dental dam frame for positioning. A dental dam napkin is a cotton sheet placed between the dam and patient to absorb moisture. A dental dam punch is a specialized type of hole puncher to tailor holes in the dental dam exactly where the teeth need to be isolated. Punches come in five ascending sizes, and are specific to the type of tooth involved:
No. 1 for mandibular incisors

No. 2 for maxillary incisors respectively
No. 3 for canines and premolars
No. 4 for molars and bridge abutments
No. 5, the largest, for the anchor tooth chosen
to hold the dental dam clamp securely

Dental dam clamps are made of stainless steel
in the shape of the crown; they come in
cervical, winged and wingless conformations,
and have a bow, jaws and forceps holes. The
dental dam forceps is for dam positioning and
removal, adding lubricant, and a dental dam
stamp. The latter is an ink-pad stamp made
like a dental arch, which serves as a guide to
indicate teeth to be punched out on the dam.

Before you insert a dental dam, the dentist
administers local anesthetic, with your help.
You must note any misaligned or malposed
teeth at this time. If a tooth is abnormally
positioned, punch holes in a corresponding
spot in the dam. Note the width of the arch
for possible accommodations. Apply
lubricant to the patient's lip with a cotton roll
or applicator. Use a mouth mirror and
explorer to find a suitable location for dam
placement. If there is any debris or plaque in
the area, brush the teeth or apply coronal
polish prior to dam positioning. Floss all
regional contacts to avoid tearing the dam.
Mark a dental dam stamp to identify the teeth
for isolation in the correct arch. Using this
template, punch the dental dam with the
correct size of dam punch. Make a hole for
the anchor and the tooth for isolation.
Lubricate holes that stretch over tight
contacts with water-soluble lubricant on the
underside.

Attach the correct clamp to both a floss safety
line and locked dental dam forceps. Fit the
dam over the anchor tooth, initially over the
lingual side. Widen your forceps, and place
the dam over the buccal side. Place the
previously punched dental dam over the
clamp bow, using your index fingers to
stretch it over the clamp and anchor tooth.
Pull the safety line to the outside. Fasten the
dam to the last tooth at the opposite end with
floss or cord. Place the dental napkin

between the outer parts of the dam and the
patient's mouth. Affix the dental dam frame
over the oral cavity to hold the dam in place.
Isolate the other teeth through the punched
holes and push them into place by using
dental floss or tape. Dry the teeth with the air
syringe. Seal all edges by tucking or inverting
them into the sulcus of the gum with a
tucking instrument, before performing the
desired procedure.

The first step of dental dam removal is to
stretch the dam material outward with your
middle or index finger. Cut each interseptal
dam. Remove the dam clamp with the dam
forceps by placing them into the forceps holes
and compressing the handles to open the
jaws of the clamp. Rotate the clamp toward
each side for easy removal. Remove the
holder, dam material, and napkin. Examine
the dam is examined to ensure no material is
left interdentally. Floss the patient's teeth, if
indicated. Knead the gum around the anchor
tooth to improve circulation. Rinse your
patient's mouth. Remove any remaining
debris.

Ultrasonic Scaler

Manual scalers have straight or curved sickles
and pointed tips at each end; they are used
most often to remove supragingival calculus.
An alternative is the ultrasonic scaler
(Cavitron), which removes heavy calculus and
stain from tooth surfaces, cement, and
bonding substances used in orthodontic
work. An ultrasonic scaler uses high-
frequency sound waves, which it translates
into mechanical energy, in the form of high-
speed vibrations at its tip. Water ejects at the
tip to control heat buildup. The combination
of vibrational energy and water facilitates
thorough removal of debris. There are
universal tips and narrower, slim line tips
available. There are also sonic scalers, which
are attached to the dental unit handpiece, and
use air to remove calculus. Both have pen-
like structures attached to their tips.

Coronal Polish

A coronal polish is a process by which soft deposits and extrinsic stains are removed from the clinical crown of teeth with abrasive material. You require a dental handpiece and a rubber cup for easiest application, but you can substitute brushes, dental tape, or floss, if necessary. Perform coronal polishing after hard deposits are scaled away. The coronal polish is performed for three main reasons:
It helps the patient maintain clean teeth and sustain good oral hygiene
The procedure enhances fluoride absorption and discourages buildup of new deposits
It prepares teeth for use of enamel sealant and for positioning of orthodontic brackets and bands
In many states, the dental assistant or hygienist can legally perform a coronal polish. If your dentist delegates polishing to you, seat yourself in the appropriate operator's position.
A coronal polish can remove soft deposits and extrinsic stains. Calculus (hardened, calcified deposits) and intrinsic stains cannot be eliminated through coronal polishing. The dentist removes calculus is prior to the polish via scaling. Intrinsic stains are within the tooth structure and are usually permanent. For example, dental fluorosis, metal poisoning, tetracycline exposure in childhood or pulp damage cannot be removed by polishing. There are four types of soft deposits removed by coronal polishing:

1. Materia alba, a less structured a precursor to plaque development, which contains microorganisms and leads to tooth decay, gingivitis and periodontal disease
2. Plaque, which contains microorganisms that damage teeth and gums
3. Food debris
4. Pellicle, a thin film containing saliva and sulcular fluid

Extrinsic stains from endogenous sources can be removed by coronal polishing. For example, yellow or brown stains associated with poor dental hygiene and tobacco can be polished away.

Abrasives are rough, particulate materials that create friction to smooth out the tooth surface during coronal polishing. Abrasives come in powder or paste form, and usually contain water, a binder, a humectant for water retention, coloring and flavoring. Available abrasive agents include fluoride pastes, flour of pumice, chalk, zirconium silicate, and tin oxide. The rate of abrasion for a particular type of abrasive is dependent upon the characteristics of the abrasive material, the speed of the handpiece, the pressure and amount applied, and the moisture level. Abrasion increases if the particles are sharp-edged, firmer, stronger, larger in size, or resist embedding in the tooth's surface.

Apply disclosing agent to teeth with a cotton applicator for easier plaque recognition.
Ask your patient if he/she is allergic to latex rubber; if yes, choose a synthetic rubber cup.
Attach a prophy cup to a low-speed dental handpiece at an angle.
Place abrasive agent into the cup; if you use more than one type, use an individual cup for each.
Hold the handpiece with cup in a modified pen grasp.
Apply foot pressure on the rheostat to regulate speed.
Polish one quadrant at a time. Position the cup near the sulcus of the gum on the mesial or distal surface of a tooth. Employ gentle pressure to bend the cup. Work toward the occlusal or incisal edge. Lift the cup a little. Duplicate the procedure on the other side of the tooth.
Frequently rinse and remove debris during the procedure.
Repeat on the adjacent tooth, until all teeth are polished.
Reapply disclosing agent to check your work. Rinse.

Prophy brushes are soft, supple brushes made of nylon or natural bristles. Perform prophy brushing after the rubber cup polish. Attach one brush to a low-speed dental handpiece. Only polish the enamel surfaces of teeth. Do not allow the brush to contact the gums. Spread prophy paste over the brush. Start polishing the most posterior tooth. For the back teeth, the major objective is to polish the occlusal surfaces. For each posterior tooth, direct the brush from the central fossa first, toward the mesial buccal cusp tip, and then toward the distal buccal cusp. For the anterior teeth, position the brush in the lingual pit above the cingulum, and then toward the incisal edge during polishing. All lingual surfaces with pits or grooves should be polished similarly. At the end, rinse your patient's mouth and clear it of debris.

After you perform a coronal polish using a prophy cup and a prophy brush, polish them interproximally with dental tape and floss. Cut a 12 to 18 inch piece of dental tape. Apply abrasive to the interproximal contact places between teeth with your finger or a cotton tip applicator. Work on one quadrant at a time. Manipulate the dental tape between your middle fingers on each hand. Insert the tape obliquely into the contact area, using a back-and-forth motion and light pressure, and then wrap the tape around the tooth. Polish the proximal surfaces of each tooth with the tape, moving along adjacent teeth. Rinse and evacuate your patient's mouth. Remove any remaining residue with dental floss and subsequently rinsing. Use unwaxed floss if the dentist will follow with a fluoride application afterwards, because waxed floss coats the teeth and deters fluoride absorption.

You require a good dental light, cheek retractors, a mouth mirror, an air-water syringe, an evacuator, a saliva ejector, and wipes to polish teeth correctly. Supplementary polishing aids that might be useful during the final phase are dental tape and floss. One aid that is useful for patients with orthodontic work is a bridge threader, a plastic piece with a loop through which dental tape or floss is passed. A threader allows the assistant to work around orthodontic or other appliances. Various grit size abrasive polishing strips can be employed on enamel facades. Soft wood points can be used with abrasives. Small interproximal brushes can be utilized. The latter are especially useful for navigation around orthodontic appliances and other contact areas.

Dental Plaque

Dental plaque is a tacky, bacteria-containing mass found on teeth that have not been brushed thoroughly. It looks like a soft, white, sticky accumulation. It is concentrated near the gingiva. The bacteria feed off consumed sugar and convert it to acid. The acid, in turn, damages the tooth enamel by causing demineralization. The content of the minerals calcium and phosphate is depressed. Demineralization on enamel surfaces looks chalky and white. Demineralization is often a problem found in patients who have had orthodontic appliances removed where the brackets were previously situated. Eventually, plaque that is not removed leads to tooth decay.

Disclosing Agents

Disclosing agents are temporary coloring agents in chewable tablet and liquid forms, usually red. Disclosing agents adhere to plaque to help the assistant and patient identify it much more easily. The assistant uses agents to check coronal polishing technique. When the dental assistant or hygienist uses disclosing agent in the office, he/she should wear Personal Protective Equipment (PPEs). Spread petroleum jelly over the patient's lips and tooth-colored restorations. Decant agent into a Dappen dish. Paint liquid agent onto the teeth with a cotton tip applicator or put it on the tongue to spread. Alternatively, ask your patient to chew a tablet and swirl it around in the mouth. Rinse and withdraw excess solution. Give the patient a hand mirror. You use a mouth mirror and air-water syringe. Chart the plaque present, using an overglove. Educate your patient education about oral hygiene. Disclosing agents encourage the patient to use good oral hygiene at home.

Fluoride

Fluoride is a mineral derivative of the element fluorine. Fluoride is primarily absorbed via the gastrointestinal tract, and is found in low amounts in normal bone and dental enamel. Fluoride incorporated into tooth enamel forms fluoroapatite crystals. Optimal fluoride exposure should be between 0.7 and 1.2 ppm, giving the teeth a gleaming, white, unblemished appearance. Average fluoride levels are lower in teeth with caries. If high amounts of fluoride are ingested during tooth development, the child's teeth acquire a mottled appearance, known as fluorosis. Excessive fluoride causes either chronic or acute fluoride poisoning. Chronic fluoride poisoning occurs from habitual ingestion, usually through a fluoridated water supply. Teeth mottle with a fluoride content up to 1.8 ppm. Enamel hypocalcifies at 1.8 to 2.0 ppm of fluoride, so teeth are chalky, with discolored bands, flecks, cracks, and pits.

Fluoride can reduce dental caries because it binds to the bacteria in plaque, thus retarding acid production and decay. Fluoride can remineralize soft areas and reverse very early tooth decay. Dentists and hygienists administer gel or foam fluoride in trays to reinforce children's teeth once or twice yearly. Topical fluoride only accesses the outer enamel layer.

Systemic Sources of Fluoride	Topical Sources of Fluoride	
Fluoridation of the water supply with 0.7 to 1.2 parts sodium fluoride per million parts water	2% Sodium fluoride	Professionally applied
Ingestion of meat, cereals, and citrus fruits	8% Stannous fluoride	
Prescription tablets, drops, lozenges, or vitamin preparations given to children up until their second molars erupt	1.23% Acidulated phosphate fluoride	
	Dentifrices (toothpastes)	Self-applied
	Polishing pastes	
	Mouth rinses	

Topical fluoride application in the dental office is usually done using 2% sodium fluoride, 8% stannous fluoride, or 1.23% acidulated phosphate fluoride (APF). Sodium fluoride preparations are stable, do not cause discoloration, and are gentle to tissues, but they must be applied weekly for four weeks each time. Stannous fluoride has many disadvantages, including instability, a caustic taste, and discoloration due to tin in the preparation. Thus, the APF preparations are used most often, as they are non-irritating, have a mild taste, do not cause discoloration, and need to be used only once or twice a year. Keep APF preparations in plastic containers to discourage acidification.

The dental assistant performs fluoride application after a rubber cup polish. Never apply fluoride before placement of orthodontic bands or sealants, as it deters adhesion. Don personal protective equipment (PPE). Select fluoride trays that encompass all erupted teeth but do not extend beyond them. Fill each tray one-third full with the fluoride gel or foam. Dry the patient's teeth with the air syringe. Position the trays in the patient's mouth and shift them up and down to distribute the fluoride preparation. Keep the saliva ejector in your patient's mouth throughout the procedure to remove saliva and moisture. Instruct the patient to keep his/her mouth closed for the recommended time. Remove the ejector trays. Evacuate the patient's mouth. Advise the patient not to eat, drink, or rinse for 30 minutes following the application. Using overgloves, chart the application and any consequences. An alternative to foam or gel application is the use of a fluoride rinse after tooth brushing or a rubber cup polish.

Retractors

Retractors redirect tissue, so the dentist sees clearly during procedures. Retractors are for oral surgery, but have other applications, too. There are tissue, cheek and lip, and tongue retractors. Tissue retractors have small jagged edges on the working end to grasp tissue, and resemble forceps or cotton pliers. Cheek and lip retractors are large metal or plastic tools that fit into the mouth to pull the cheeks or lips outward, expanding the viewing region. Tongue retractors are spoon-shaped or lengthy blades that displace the tongue. Place tongue retractors between the rim of the tongue and the lingual surfaces of the teeth, or adapt them for cheek retraction by positioning them on the buccal mucosa. Hemostats and needle holders are forceps with jagged beaks and locking handles, usable for retraction. Insert mouth props when the patient's mouth must be open for a long period. They are stainless steel, silicone, plastic, or hard rubber, and come in various sizes. The locking Molt mouth gag is an example.

Patient Management

Psychology is the study of the mind and people's characteristic mental makeup. Each person brings an acquired belief system (paradigm) to his/her interactions with others. Patients have preconceived ideas about dental practices. Many are apprehensive about pain. The dental assistant must understand paradigms and employ good communication and listening skills to facilitate successful patient interaction and management. Communication is the exchange of information. Good communication consists of skillful interpretation of the message by the sender (in this case the dental professional), interpretation of the message by the receiver (the patient), and establishment of a connection, as indicated by feedback. Active listening on the part of both sender and receiver enhances good communication.

Any type of communication between people that does not involve words is non-verbal communication. Up to 93% of successful communication depends on nonverbal cues. Remember that a dental patient is unable to speak during a procedure and is likely apprehensive. Watch your patient's facial expressions, gestures, posture, and position. Tight posture and/or crossed arms and legs suggest resistance. Conversely, relaxed posture and uncrossed appendage suggest openness. Your posture affects your patient. Sit close to your patient, rather than towering directly over him/her in an intimidating manner. Maintain the proper social distance (territoriality) between yourself and your patient during discussions (~3 feet). A patient feels more comfortable when he/she is well-informed beforehand and the professional works from the side.

Different cultures have different value systems, and the dental professional must be aware of these to ensure a successful practice. Realize that social distance, eye contact, and use of first names versus surnames differs among cultures. For example: Arabs find a social distance of 2 feet best; Asians find direct eye contact rude; Israelis talk on a first-name basis; and in Hispanic cultures, the oldest male family member speaks for the patient. Familiarize yourself with the

- 32 -

immigrant population in your area and take diversity training. The American Dental Association offers Spanish explanations of common procedures at http://www.ada.org/public/espanol/index.asp. Know where you can find interpreters who understand dental terminology. Book the interpreter at least a day before the procedure. Speak slowly while facing the patient; do not address the translator first. Try to get more than perfunctory feedback from the patient during the communication.

Pain and Anxiety Control

Before, during and/or after dental procedures, the dentist administers some type of pain and anxiety control to the patient. The dental assistant preps the supplies. The dentist can alleviate pain and anxiety by psychological methods, such as hypnosis and biofeedback, by chemicals, or by physiologic agents. The dentist can prescribe five types of pain relief:
1. Antianxiety drugs that relieve apprehension (e.g., Valium)
2. Local or topical anesthetic that dulls pain (e.g., lidocaine)
3. Inhalation sedation that induces a state of calm drowsiness (e.g., nitrous oxide N_2O)
4. Intravenous sedation (e.g., Versed, a benzodiazepine)
5. General anesthesia by Jorgensen technique, which induces unconsciousness (e.g., pentobarbital sodium, a barbiturate, mixed with Demerol, an opioids, and scopolamine, an anticholinergic)

Topical and Local Anesthetics

All anesthetics block nerve impulses, thus dulling pain sensations. The dentist or nurse spreads topical anesthetic directly over oral mucosa before injecting a local anesthetic. Topical preparations are usually ointments applied with a cotton swab, but they can be sprays, liquids, and patches. Local anesthetics are chemical amides and esters, and are injected in the proximity of the nerve associated with the tooth being treated. Local anesthetic agents have a particular timeframe after injection for induction of full numbing and later loss of numbing (duration). Local anesthetics are classified in terms of their duration as short-acting, intermediate-acting, or long-acting. Most procedures require the intermediate-acting duration of 2 to 4 hours. Most intermediate-acting and long-acting local anesthetic agents also contain small concentrations of vasoconstrictors, such as epinephrine, which decrease blood flow and bleeding to the region. These preparations are contraindicated in patients with hypertension, cardiovascular disease, liver or kidney disease, hyperthyroidism, or pregnancy.

Local anesthesia methods fall into 3 categories:

Local infiltration — The dentist injects the agent into gingival tissues near the small terminal nerve branches, numbing the necessary tooth and/or gums. The anesthetic can also be injected using pressure right into the periodontal ligament.

Field block — The dentist injects the agent at the larger terminal nerve limbs near the apex of the tooth. The advantages of field block technique are avoidance of messages to the central nervous system and swift onset of action.

Nerve block — The dentist introduces the agent close to a main nerve trunk, which eliminates pain sensations to the brain, and over a relatively large local area.

Local infiltration or field block techniques desensitize individual maxillary teeth when injected near the apex of specific anterior teeth. A nasopalatine nerve block, in which the lingual tissue next to the incisive papilla is injected, numbs the front of the hard palate between the canines. The greater palatine nerve block uses injection near the second molar and in front of the greater palatine foramen to block sensations to the entire hard palate and soft tissues posterior to the canine. A maxillary nerve block is an anesthetic injection into the mucobuccal fold near the second molar, which blocks one entire oral quadrant, and the skin on that side of the nose, cheek, upper lip and lower eyelid. The anterior superior alveolar, middle superior alveolar, and posterior superior alveolar nerve blocks involve injection into the fold at the first premolar, fold at the second premolar, and near the apex of the second molar respectively; each affects two or three close teeth and tissues.

Local infiltration or field block techniques desensitize individual mandibular teeth by injecting near the apex of specific anterior teeth. Nerve blocks numb larger areas. Introduction of anesthetic into the mucobuccal fold in front of the mental foramen is an incisive nerve block, affecting teeth from the central incisors back to the premolars and the cheeks. Inferior alveolar nerve block or mandibular block dulls an entire quadrant, including teeth, mucous membranes, the front portion of the tongue, mouth floor, and soft tissues. It involves injection into the mandibular ramus, behind the retromolar pad. Lingual nerve block means the anesthetic is introduced lingually to the mandibular ramus and next to the maxillary tuberosity, affecting the mandibular teeth, the side of the tongue, and lingual tissues on one side. Buccal nerve block means the agent is injected into the mucous membrane behind the last available molar just to numb buccal tissue. Mental nerve block involves an injection between the apices of the premolars, to target the premolars, canines, and close facial tissues.

Anesthetic Syringe

An anesthetic or aspirating syringe consists of the barrel, the disposable needle cannula, and the anesthetic cartridge. Both reusable stainless steel and disposable plastic syringes are available. The operator braces the thumb in a ring at one end and the index and middle fingers on grips. The barrel of the syringe is a long shaft, open on one side for cartridge insertion, with an observation window on the opposite side. Inside the barrel is a plunger or piston rod attached to a barbed-tipped harpoon at its end. There is a threaded tip at the end of the syringe, to which the sterile disposable needle (cannula) is attached. The cannula has a short cartridge end attached to needle hub, which is either pushed or screwed onto the threaded tip of the syringe. The slanted tip (bevel) on the other end penetrates tissue. The segment between is the shank; the solution travels through its internal, hollow lumen. Anesthetic cartridges containing the agent are made of glass. They have a rubber stopper end to attach to the harpoon of the syringe and an aluminum cap end for needle insertion.

Anesthetic cartridges labeled with the American Dental Association's seal of acceptance have standardized color codes on a band near the rubber stopper. Sometimes, the aluminum cap is also colored similarly, although it may be silver. There is unambiguous, black lettering on the cartridge, identifying the agent and concentration. Some other cartridges have colored writing on the side. The ADA-approved color schemes are as follows:

Articaine 4% with epinephrine 1:100,000 – gold

Bupivacaine with epinephrine – blue

Lidocaine 2% either plain or with epinephrine 1:50,000 or 1:100,000 - light blue, green, or red, respectively

Mepivacaine 3% or 2% with levonordefrin 1:20,000 - tan or brown, respectively

Prilocaine 4% without or with epinephrine 1:200,000 - black or yellow, respectively

Sanitize the harpoon of a stainless steel reusable aspirating syringe after each use and autoclave the entire syringe. From time to time, lubricate parts or the harpoon may require exchange. Discard plastic syringes in a biohazard container. Discard the cannula into a sharps container after normal use, if there is any evidence of a broken seal, or if tissue penetration occurs more than four times. Anesthetic cartridges come in sterilized, sealed blister packs and should be stored at room temperature in a dark area. Inspect the cartridge before use. Discard a cartridge that has expired or has large bubbles, rust, corrosion, or extruded stoppers. Dispose of a used cartridge in a tamper-proof container approved by the pharmacist. Be aware that addicts scavenge garbage for residual drugs.

The dental assistant is responsible for preparation of the anesthetic syringe outside the viewing area of the patient. Take the sterile syringe out of its autoclave pouch. Hold the syringe in your left hand. Withdraw the piston rod by pulling back on the thumb ring. With your right hand, position the rubber stopper end of the cartridge into the barrel of the syringe. Connect he harpoon to the rubber stopper using medium pressure on the finger ring. Take off the cap of the syringe end of the disposable needle and screw or push it onto the threaded tip of the syringe. Remove the needle guard. Check for correct operation by forcing out a small amount of reagent, while holding the syringe upright.

The assistant prepares local anesthetic. The dentist dries the injection site with a sterile gauze sponge and applies topical anesthetic with a cotton swab for one minute. The assistant transfers the syringe to the dentist, either beneath the patient's chin or behind the patient's head. Pass the syringe with the thumb ring toward the dentist, the bevel of the needle facing the alveolar bone, and the protective cap secure but loose enough to remove during the transfer. The dentist performs the injection. The assistant observes the patient for adverse reactions. The dentist replaces the needle guard by scooping or uses a mechanical recapping device. If the patient requires additional anesthesia, the assistant swaps in a new cartridge and transfers it, as above. Replace the recapped syringe on the tray. Rinse and evacuate the patient's mouth at the conclusion of the procedure. Remove the capped needle by unscrewing or cutting it off and discarding it in the sharps container. Remove the cartridge by retraction of the piston and deposit it in a medical waste container. Sterilize the syringe.

One relatively painless and fast method is intraosseous anesthesia, in which the cortical plate of bone is first perforated using a solid needle connected to a slow handpiece. The anesthetic agent is then injected into the hole, using an 8 mm, 27-gauge needle. Periodontal ligament injection entails insertion into the gingival sulcus. A special injection syringe is used; it is gun-like and the syringe is attached externally. Another technique is intrapulpal injection right into the pulp chamber or root canal, using a 25-gauge or 27-gauge needle. There are computer operated delivery systems available for administration of local anesthesia, which offer the ability to control parameters, such as rate of delivery and pressure. There are also systems that deliver electronic impulses, instead of chemical preparations, in cases where chemicals are contraindicated.

Nitrous Oxide

Analgesics are agents that relieve pain without loss of consciousness. Nitrous oxide (N_2O) is an analgesic dispensed simultaneously with oxygen (O_2) gas through a small nosepiece, connected via tubing to a tank. The inhaled gases migrate through the nasopharynx, the respiratory chambers, and eventually reach the alveoli in the lungs. The gasses are exchanged between the alveoli and the blood plasma and red cells. The circulatory system transports the gases by the blood to the brain, where the analgesic effect is initiated. Nitrous oxide and oxygen together have mild pharmacologic activity in the central nervous system. They create a state of calmness for the patient, called sedation. The setup generally includes an inside mask for inhalation of the gases, an outer mask attached to an external reservoir bag, and a vacuum to carry away exhaled and excess gas.

The American Dental Association suggests that personnel in dental offices who administer nitrous oxide be monitored twice a year by dosimetry or infrared spectrophotometry. Nitrous oxide is associated with infertility problems.

DO NOT administer nitrous oxide to:	Use Nitrous Oxide for:
Pregnant women in the first trimester	Apprehensive patients
Infertile individuals undergoing in-vitro fertilization procedures	Patient with sensitive gag reflexes
Neurology patients	Heart patients, who benefit from The latter benefit from supplemental oxygen and reduction of stress
Drug abusers	
Psychiatric patients	
Immunocompromised patients in danger of bone marrow suppression	
Mouth breathers	Nose breathers

Depending on the state, these functions may be done by the dental assistant under supervision of the dentist, or as a cooperative effort. The assistant is responsible for rechecking equipment, gas levels in the tanks, and preparing the patient. The dentist explains the procedure and hazards involved to the patient. Ask the patient to sign an informed consent form. Tilt the patient back in the chair. Attach a sterile nitrous mask to the tubing. Connect it to the tanks. Place the mask over the patient's nose. Tell the patient to breathe slowly through his/her nose. When indicated by the dentist, administer oxygen alone for one minute, at a rate of at least 5 liters per minute, to determine the

normal tidal volume. Administer nitrous oxide in 500 ml to 1 liter increments per minute, with equivalent reduction of oxygen flow. Observe patient response to determine the optimal mixture that provides sedation, without impeding cognition. The dentist gives local anesthetic a few minutes after nitrous oxide administration is initiated.

Turn off the nitrous oxide under the dentist's direction. Allow the patient to receive only oxygen for about 5 minutes to stave off diffusion hypoxia, the inadequate supply of oxygen to bodily tissues. Remove the patient's mask. Tilt the chair upright to avoid postural hypotension or fainting. Do not dismiss the patient until he/she feels clear-headed (usually a few minutes). Chart the nitrous oxide administration, including baseline levels of both gases, and the patient's reactions. A good method of judging the psychomotor ability of the patient is to give a Trieger test prior to administration and after recovery. The Trieger test involves connecting a pattern of dots. The patient completes the test in the upright position. Disinfect the connecting tubing after use. Depending on office procedures, the masks may be discarded, or given to the patient for later reuse.

Routine Prophylaxis

Dental prophylaxis means preventing dental disease by identifying and removing plaque and debris from tooth surfaces. The armamentarium suggested for routine prophylaxis consists of various sickle scalers, a universal curette, an explorer, floss, a saliva ejector and HVE tip, a Dappen dish, disclosing solution, air and water syringe tips, cotton swabs, gauze sponges, prophy paste, and angle and ring holders. If root planing or smoothing is to be performed, include several Gracey curettes and a setup for local anesthesia, including the anesthetic.

Scalers are hand-held instruments that remove undesirable substances from tooth surfaces. Most scalers used for routine prophylaxis are either sickle or curette scalers. Sickle scalers have long tapered tips with pointed toes. They are suitable for scaling under interproximal contact areas in the front of the mouth. Common sickle scalers include single-ended and double-ended straight sickles and a curved straight sickle (usually two or more curved cutting edges). Curette scalers, can scale all tooth surfaces and are especially useful for removing subgingival calculus and root planing. They have rounded tips and backs and cutting edges. A universal curette is often employed for routine prophylaxis. It is straight and the entire edge is used to cut. Gracey curettes are designed to scale specific tooth surfaces or for root planing. They are curved at the end and only one side and the tip are used to cut. Gracey curettes are designated by their angles at either end, ranging from 1 for anterior teeth to 16 for posterior teeth surfaces. Dental explorers have very fine tips. They are used to check for calculus in subgingival regions during scaling.

Routine dental prophylaxis consists of an assessment and a treatment phase. During the assessment phase, the assistant applies disclosing agent to the patient's teeth to identify plaque accumulation. The treatment phase has four parts:

Scaling or scraping off undesirable substances on the surfaces of teeth, such as hard calculus and softer plaque with various scalers, and using the explorer to check subgingival portions. The dental assistant aids the dentist by using the oral evacuator or gauze sponges. Root planing may be performed now or scheduled separately.

Coronal polishing is performed with a dental handpiece and prophy paste or an air-powder abrasive polisher, to remove further plaque and stains and leave a smooth surface. Again the assistant aids with evacuation.

Flossing is performed to guarantee plaque removal between teeth.

Fluoride treatment is an elective procedure.

Dental Handpieces

The dental unit is the center from which dental handpieces and other essential equipment, such as the oral evacuator and air-water syringe, are controlled. The unit is set up to deliver instruments to the dentist from the rear, on the side of the dentist, or transthorax (over the patient's chest). There are at least two high-speed and one slow speed handpiece and an air-water syringe connected to the unit. Slow-speed handpieces are straight and are used for decay removal, fine finishing, and polishing. Accessories are attached to the end, depending on the intended use. Slightly bent contra-angle attachments hold either friction-grip (FG) or latch-type (RA) burrs. The prophylaxis angle holds the polishing cup or brush. Low-torque, high-speed handpieces have curved ends. They are used with hard carbon steel burrs or diamond stones to remove the greater part of tooth structure for restoration before refinement. The friction generated necessitates use of a cooling water spray. The assistant is responsible for evacuation.

A burr is a tool attached to the end of a handpiece to remove rough edges of tooth structure. They are composed of stainless steel, or carbide metal, or diamond chips. The shanks to which the head (working end) and neck are attached are either friction-grip (FG), latch-type (RA), or straight handpiece (HP) types. There are a variety of types of slow-speed burrs, including:

- Acrylic burrs (used for acrylic-based dentures or orthodontic appliances)
- Straight HP finishing burrs (principally utilized for finishing gold, amalgam or composite restorations)
- Diamond stones (used for crown preparation)
- Green stones (for finishing gold, amalgam or composite restorations)

- Acrylic stones (again for acrylic dentures and orthodontic appliances)
- A mandrel or shaft can be connect to the handpiece and attached to sandpaper or abrasive discs with diamond or carborundum grit for finishing functions, or a bristle brush for tooth polishing.

High-speed handpieces are principally used to remove undesired tooth structure swiftly, before finishing procedures. Therefore, burrs used with high-speed handpieces are made of carbon steel or diamond stones. Caries removal requires either round burrs or inverted cones. Round burrs open the pulp chamber for a root canal. Inverted cones are used for cavity preparation. Fissure burrs have flat ends and regularly spaced lines around the shaft. The straight fissure burrs, either plain cut or crosscut, make the initial opening into a tooth for smoothing the walls of a cavity or for axial retention grooves. The tapered versions are for inlay preparations or to open the pulp chamber for a root canal. Finishing burrs can be round, oval, pear or flame shaped. They are for finer aspects of amalgam or composite restorations. Wheel burrs form retentions. End cutting burrs form the shoulder for crowns. Burrs are numbered to reflect their shape, size and differences.

Hand Cutting Instruments

Prior to use of handpieces, hand cutting instruments were used to prepare cavities. Now, hand instruments are for fine detailing. They consist of a central shaft or handle connected to shanks on one or both ends, attached to a bevel and some type of working end, usually a blade and cutting edge. The hand instrument is described in terms of its shank angles (e.g., straight, slightly curved or Wedelstaedt, monangle, binangle, and triple angle) and the class of cutting edge. There are five common classes of cutting edge: Hatchet, chisel, hoe, margin trimmer, and angle former. Both hatchets and hoes plane cavity walls and floors. The dentist uses a pulling motion. Hatchets and angle formers hone angles. Chisels are used with a pulling motion to plane enamel margins and to trim margins on front teeth. Special gingival angle formers (gingival margin trimmers), which have curved working ends, shape the cervical cavosurface margin in amalgam and inlay restorations. Excavators have more rounded blades to extract decay and debris.

Black's Formula

G. V. Black invented a formula to describe hand cutting instruments in terms of the size of the blade and its angle relative to the shaft. There are two different formulae, a 3-number and a 4-number. The Black's Three Number Formula describes chisels, hatchets, and hoes. It consists of the first number for the width of the blade in tenths of a millimeter, the second number for the blade's length in millimeters, and the third number for the angle between the blade and the long axis of the shaft in degrees centigrade (parts per hundred of a complete circle). Thus, a blade designated as (18 8 15) is 1.8 mm wide, 8 mm long, and at an angle of 15/100 of a circle to the handle. The Black's Four Number Formula describes angle formers and gingival margin trimmers. Its first, third, and fourth number correspond to the same descriptions as the first, second and third numbers in the Three Number Formula. The fourth number represents the angle of the cutting edge relative to the handle.

Non-Cutting Hand Instruments

Hand instruments not used for cutting fall into two classifications: Those used for basic examinations and those used to finish amalgam and composite restorative materials. Non-cutting instruments have configurations similar to cutting ones (handle, shank, and working end). Basic examination implements include mouth mirrors, explorers, cotton pliers, and periodontal probes. Categories of mouth mirrors include plane or regular with silver coatings on the glass back, front surface mirrors with rhodium on the front of the glass, and concave surface mirrors for magnification. The working end(s) of explorers are thin for probing; common configurations are the pigtail and shepherd's hook. Cotton pliers, which resemble large tweezers, transfer cotton rolls and other materials. Periodontal probes have round or blunt working ends and gauge the depth of the gingival sulcus.

Non-cutting hand instruments that are used for finishing restorative materials include filling instruments, amalgam carriers, amalgam condensers, carvers, burnishers, files, and finishing knives. Most have the same basic configuration of handle, shank and working end. Filling instruments, which put restorative materials and cement bases into the cavity preparation, are thermoplastic or anodized aluminum. Hand amalgam condensers (pluggers) press amalgam into the cavity preparation; there are also mechanical vibrating versions. Carvers are designed with working ends that can get rid of excess restorative agents or carve tooth anatomy; they are generally used on crowns, inlays and onlays. Burnishers smooth coarse margins or shape matrix bands. Both files and finishing knives, which have sharper ends, trim excess filling materials. Amalgam carriers load and place the amalgam; there are amalgam guns for composites, glass ionomers and alloys.

Miscellaneous Hand Instruments

Miscellaneous hand implements for restorations include spatulas, articulating forceps, and scissors. The commonly used spatulas are stainless steel cement spatulas for mixing cements and other materials, plastic for mixing composite resins, and larger general laboratory spatulas for blending impression materials or plaster. Articulating forceps grasp articulation paper (special heavy paper showing marks if contact is made) for checking occlusion after adding the restorative material. The type of scissor used most often for restorations is the crown and collar scissors (also called the bridge scissors), which have short straight or curved cutting blades. Scissors cut retraction cords and trim matrix bands.

Cavity Preparation

Cavity preparation is the orderly cutting of tooth structure to remove any undesired portions, such decay, pits or fissures susceptible to caries, fractured tooth fragments, or enamel without underlying dentin support. The four steps of cavity preparation are:
1. Opening up the cavity with a burr
2. Outlining
3. Refining
4. Finishing it with other instruments

The dentist considers three and sometimes four factors when preparing a cavity. The first is the outline form or general shape of the preparation, which depends on the amount of decay, the material to be used, and how it can be retained. The resistance form is the internal contour of the cavity preparation. The dentist takes into account potential biting forces. The retention form is the internal profile of the cavity walls needed to keep the restoration in place, for example, using retention grooves or undercutting. There can also be a convenience form, which may be slightly larger than the outline form, to allow for use of instrumentation.

Cavity preparation creates walls, lines and angles within the tooth. Walls are any side or floor of the preparation. They are described in terms of the nearest tooth surface, for example distal, buccal, pulpal (over the pulp), axial (parallel to the tooth's long axis), or gingival (perpendicular to the long axis). Lines are created when two surfaces converge. Preparation is described in terms of the line angles that result, for example, the buccopulpal line angle or mesiobuccal line angle. When three surfaces converge, they form point angles, for example, the mesiobuccopulpal point angle or distobuccopulpal point angle. Another angle is the cavosurface margin, which is the angle between the preparation and untouched tooth surface; it is important to seal these surfaces. In any cavity preparation, there are numerous line and point angles. Cavities are described in terms of depth. An ideal depth is shallow enough to retain the restorative material, a moderate depth is a slightly deeper one that does not invade the pulp, and a very deep preparation very nearly or actually exposes pulp.

The dentist cleans the cavity and usually medicates it prior to inserting the restoration. Medication ensures maintenance of healthy pulp because it:

- Seals dentin tubules
- Calms pulpal irritation
- Stimulates pulp healing
- Provides a barrier between dentin and the restoration material for thermal insulation or to discharge fluoride into the area

Three substances are used for medication: Thin, creamy cavity liners, like calcium hydroxide or glass ionomer; or cavity varnish; or cement bases, which include glass ionomer, zinc oxide and eugenol, and zinc phosphate. Suggested medication procedures depend on the restoration material and the depth of the cavity's preparation. For ideal depth cavity preparations, rinse the tooth and dry it with the air-water syringe.

Metal amalgam restorations require either two thin coats of cavity varnish or one of glass ionomer placed over the exposed dentin. Glass ionomer is recommended for composite or acrylic restorations. These are cavity liners. If the cavity preparation is of moderate depth, a cavity liner is also sufficient for amalgam restorations. Glass ionomer liners are suggested for composite restorations. Very deep cavity preparations require more extensive medication techniques. For amalgam restorations, usually the dentist applies calcium hydroxide to the deepest part then a cement base, and finally, two layers of cavity varnish. For composite restorations, an initial calcium hydroxide liner in the deepest portion should be followed by a glass ionomer base before the composite is added.

Amalgam

Amalgam is an alloy, a mixture of metals or metal and some nonmetallic material. Dental amalgam consists of silver, tin, copper and sometimes zinc which is then mixed with mercury. Unalloyed liquid mercury is a neurotoxin; treat it as a hazardous material. The way in which the dental alloy portion of the amalgam was prepared affects its properties, especially the relative concentration of components and the shape of copper particles. The major component (40% to 70%) of dental alloys is silver, which combines with the mercury to form a compound that eventually hardens. Tin, found in concentrations from about 22% to 37%, has a strong affinity for mercury and encourages the amalgamation. Copper increases the strength and hardness of the amalgam. Amalgams are usually defined as low copper (4% to 5%) or high copper (12% to 30 %), with the latter providing strength and corrosion resistance. Zinc may be added in small concentrations up to 1% to minimize the oxidation of the other metals.

Amalgam is supplied in color-coded capsules containing premeasured amounts of silver alloy powder and mercury. The color indicates whether the amount of material is appropriate for small cavity preparations (a single spill), or for larger cavities (double or triple spills). A metal or plastic pestle is provided for mixing the two ingredients when the capsule is opened. An amalgamator is an instrument for mixing and initiating the amalgamation (chemical reaction) between alloy and mercury. The success of this mixing procedure, also called trituration, depends on mixing time, speed of mixing, and force applied. Larger amounts must be mixed longer. The dental assistant prepares the capsule (twist-off cap, squeezing, or using an activator), puts it into the amalgamator, mixes it as determined, and after removal empties it into a container (Dappen dish or amalgam well).

Amalgam carriers hold the amalgam and its pistons push amalgam into the site. Amalgam condensers are hand instruments with flat working ends that push the amalgam against surfaces of the cavity preparation. There are also automatic versions. Matrix bans are strips of thin stainless steel, used to fashion an outline around a prepared tooth. They are only necessary for restorations where tooth structure is lacking (class II, III and VI). The dentist uses the matrix band in parts to support condensation (pressing the amalgam into place). The matrix band is removed at the end of the restoration. A matrix retainer holds the two ends of the matrix band in place. A contouring plier shapes the matrix band. Interproximal wedges are three-sided wooden or plastic sticks that fit between the teeth after matrix band placement. Wedges prevent amalgam leakage into the interproximal space and keep adjacent teeth slightly apart. One wedge is needed for class II and III restorations. Two wedges are necessary for class IV and larger.

Tofflemire Matrix

The Tofflemire matrix assembly is the most widely-used matrix retainer for amalgam restorations. The central frame is connected at one end to a clamp-like vise. The vise has a diagonal slot through it, to grip the ends of the matrix band. Guide slots orient the matrix band loop in the correct direction. A screw-like spindle is connected to the vise and fixes the bands in place. At the opposite end is the outer adjustment knob, which is used to tighten the spindle alongside the band. Internal to that is an inner knob, which slides, and can be used for adjustment. Tofflemire setups are viewed from a gingival or an occlusal aspect, meaning the diagonal and guide slots are or are not visible respectively.

Hold the Tofflemire assembly in your left hand in a gingival aspect (slots toward the dental assistant or operator). Turn the outer knob clockwise until the spindle can be seen in the diagonal slot of the vise. Turn the inner knob until the vise is about 3/16 inch from the guide slots. Turn the outer knob counterclockwise, so the spindle is not visible in the diagonal slot. The dental assistant takes a matrix band, forming it first into a "smile" and then a loop. The occlusal edge makes the outer edge of the "smile". Insert the ends of the matrix band into the diagonal slot (occlusal edge on the bottom), while simultaneously threading the area closer to the loop into the guide slots. If the matrix band is for a tooth in the lower left or upper right quadrants, position the loop above the retainer. If the band is to for a tooth in the lower right or upper left quadrant, face the loop downward. Secure the band by turning the outer knob clockwise. Adjust the loop size with the inner knob. The shape can be rounded by using the handle of a mouth mirror.

Place the Tofflemire matrix over the prepared tooth. The correct placement is with the smaller edge of the band toward the gums, the diagonal slot toward the gingiva, and the apparatus parallel to the buccal surface. Push the band loop through the interproximal surface. Center it on the buccal surface of the tooth. Tighten the using the inner knob of the Tofflemire apparatus. Check the margins between the matrix band and cavity preparation to ensure that the band is not too tight or loose; they should be approximately 1.0 to 1.5 mm at the gingival edge and a maximum of 2 mm at the occlusal edge. Use a ball burnisher to contour the band, so there is contact with contiguous teeth. Place interproximal wedges at the gingival margins. Check with an explorer to ensure there are no gaps. After the dentist performs the restoration, remove the wedge(s) with cotton pliers or a hemostat. Loosen the retainer with the outer knob. Lift it off. Remove the matrix band with cotton pliers.

Other Apparatuses

The main apparatuses other than the Tofflemire are the AutoMatrix, the plastic strip matrix, and sectional matrix systems. The AutoMatrix apparatus is convenient because it does not use a retainer. It comes with several sizes of conical bands that have tightening coils on the exterior for adjustment. Plastic strip matrix systems use thin, transparent strips, which are placed between the teeth, then around the preparation, and secured with a wedge. Secure the strip further after the restorative materials (not amalgam) are placed by pulling tightly and holding on or using a clip retainer. Plastic strips allow polymerizing light through. A variation is a crown matrix form, used for crowns on front teeth. Sectional matrix systems are comprised of relatively thick, contoured, oval matrix bands and rings to hold them. A discrete matrix band/ring pair is used for each tooth surface. Forceps are provided to open the rings. Wedges are put in between placement of the bands to position the rings. For pediatric patients, brass straight or curved T-bands or spot-welded matrix bands may be used.

Class II Amalgam Restoration

Class II assumes an expanded role for the dental assistant, working in conjunction with the dentist. Dry the injection site. Apply topical anesthetic. Convey the mirror, explorer, gauze, and a syringe filled with local anesthetic. The dentist injects the anesthetic. The assistant rinses and evacuates. Help the dentist as needed with placement of a rubber dam. Transfer the high-speed handpiece with burr and the mouth mirror to the dentist for inserting the amalgam restoration. Retract the cheek and tongue. Keep the mirror clear with the air-water syringe. Evacuate as needed with the HVE. Transmit and receive instruments, as requested. After the preparation, clean the tooth with a cotton pellet (rinsed and dried). Prepare and transfer to the dentist on cue the cavity liner, the cavity varnish, and the base. If light curing is required, direct the light tip. Assemble the matrix retainer and band apparatus. Hand it to the dentist in the correct orientation for placement. Transfer a wedge with cotton pliers or a hemostat. When the dentist indicates readiness, prepare the amalgam and activate it (twisting, squeezing, or putting in an activator). Mix in the amalgamator. Place the mixed amalgam into an amalgam well or Dappen dish. Load it into the amalgam carrier. Alternate placement of amalgam into the cavity preparation with packing with a condenser, until the cavity is filled. Amalgam may be placed by the dentist or assistant, but the condensing is a function of the dentist alone. When the filling is complete, the assistant transfers an explorer to the dentist for releasing amalgam from the matrix bind, cleans up amalgam fragments and puts them in a sealed container, and then hands carving, finishing, and band removal instruments as requested, while evacuating with the HVE. Remove the rubber dam. Dry the site. Use articulation paper to check occlusion before cleaning off the patient. Instruct the patient not to chew on the filled side for several hours.

Pin-Retained Amalgam Restorations

Pin-retained amalgam restorations may be used for teeth with extensive damage. After the cavity has been prepared, the dentist makes starter holes where needed. The dentist drills further between the pulp and external part of the root, using a unique twist drill. The dentist screws threaded pins into the holes with an autoclutch handpiece or a tiny hand wrench. Then the matrix band and retainer are positioned. The amalgam is added and condensed around the retention pins. The band is removed after hardening. Carving and finishing are performed as usual. Retention pins can also be used to make a central amalgam core, over which a cast gold crown is placed.

Mercury Precautions

Mercury is toxic to nerves. It is liquid at room temperature and can vaporize. Take precautions at every step where exposure might occur. Follow the American Dental Association's guidelines for mercury use in the dental office. Wear disposable gloves, a face mask, and goggles when working with amalgam. Use premeasured capsules. Triturate in an amalgamator with a protective cover. Do not touch mercury with bare skin. If contact occurs, wash with soap and water and rinse well. Handle mercury only over impermeable surfaces and away from heat sources, like autoclaves. Do not eat or drink near mercury. Use a water spray, high-volume evacuation, and a mask when cutting or polishing amalgam. Store amalgam scraps and mercury in capped, unbreakable jars before disposal as hazardous waste. Properly ventilate the office. Carpet is not appropriate flooring. Educate all staff about regular urinalyses and monitoring devices for mercury. A mercury spill kit must be available.

Composite Restorations

When restorations use composite resins or glass ionomers, a filling instrument places the material in the cavity preparation. Long plastic or Teflon-tipped filling instruments are available, but usually a pistol grip composite syringe (with inserted cartridge) is used, so injection can be slowly controlled. Clear matrix strips and clamp-like strip holders retain the material. Usually, a surgical scalpel finishes composite restorations. A slow-speed handpiece may be used with various finishing stones and/or sandpaper finishing discs attached via a mandrel for polishing and contouring. These instruments need a water-soluble lubricant to reduce heat and clogging. There are special polishing strips for interproximal areas inaccessible to discs; use them like dental floss. Crown restorations require celluloid crown forms filled with composite or acrylic,

positioned over the prepared tooth until hardened, which are then discarded.

Class II Composite Restoration

Dentist's Tasks:
Injects local anesthetic
Selects the shade of composite material that matches the patient's teeth
Prepares the cavity
Applies acid etchant
Positions celluloid matrix strips, plastic wedges, and sometimes a primer
Adds composite incrementally with a filling instrument, followed by light curing or chemical self-curing
Tests the restoration with an explorer
Finishes restoration with a low-speed handpiece and abrasive attachments

Assistant's Tasks:
Rinses and dries the site
Applies topical anesthetic
Inserts a rubber dam to isolate the tooth
Keeps the area clear and evacuates it
Dries the preparation
Prepares the calcium hydroxide and/or glass ionomer base or liner for cavity medication and may light cure it
Rinses acid etchant
Mixes bonding agent, applies it, and light cures it
Holds the matrix tightly to maintain contours
Removes matrix strip, wedge, and dental dam
Examines the site, dries, and rinses it

Other Composite Restorations

Composite restorations are called aesthetic because they are tooth-colored. Increasingly, composite restorations are being used for posterior teeth, even though they are grinding surfaces. Composites are appropriate for class III , IV, and V cavity preparations. Class IV composite restorations differ from class III in these respects:
Pins are needed for retention in the cavity preparation

A cut-off portion of a celluloid crown form may be used to shape proximal and incisal portions
A celluloid crown form is used for composite insertion.
Class V preparations are usually easily filled with composite or glass ionomer, without matrix bands, and require minimal finishing. If the root surfaces are exposed, the tooth is conditioned with 10% polycyclic acid, the preparation is rinsed and dried, a calcium liner may be used, and then the composite or glass ionomer material is inserted.

Composite Resin Inlays

Composite resin inlays can be used for posterior restorations. Alternatives are gold or porcelain inlays. The dentist makes a replica or die of the tooth. The dental laboratory makes the inlay (which has high amounts of filler for strength). At the time of cementation, the dentist applies acid etchant to the prepared tooth, then bonding resin, followed by composite cement applied to the etched enamel and the interior of the inlay. The composite cement is a dual-cure bond agent because it has elements that need to be both light-cured and chemically-cured. The inlay is then placed into the cavity preparation, light cured, and attuned for margins and occlusion.

Direct Composite Veneers

Veneers are thin layers of tooth-colored materials that are bonded to the enamel surface of teeth for aesthetic reasons, such as reshaping, concealing stains, or disguising diastema (large spaces between adjacent teeth). Before any type of veneering, the assistant polishes the teeth with pumice and water. There are both direct and indirect resin veneers. Direct veneers are made in one sitting. The dentist etches the teeth with phosphoric acid gel and applies two coats of bonding resin to the etched portions. Matrix strips are used if needed. Then the dentist applies composite resin in layers, followed by light curing and shaping. Opaquers and body shades may also be used before contouring and finishing is performed.

Indirect Composite Veneers

For indirect veneers, the dentist takes an impression at the first sitting. The laboratory fabricates the veneers, which are bonded at another appointment. The dentist applies a priming agent followed by a bonding agent (without light curing) to the tooth side of the veneer. The dentist places the veneer and checks for the shade of bond agent until the correct one is found, then temporarily removes it. The assistant installs matrix strips on either side of the tooth to be veneered. The dentist acid etches it, applies bonding agent to both the etched enamel and the tooth side of the veneer, and sets the veneer. Excess bonding agent is removed by the dentist. The assistant light cures the site for about a minute before the dentist finishes it. Indirect composite veneers are not as strong as porcelain veneers.

Etched Porcelain Veneers

Etched porcelain veneers are very strong, and desirable for aesthetic restorations of upper teeth. The dentist:
Uses a diamond stone with a high-speed handpiece to take off some of the labial enamel (a retraction cord may be used)

Takes a polysiloxane or polyether impression, makes a stone model, and sends it to the dental ceramist, who makes the veneers and etches them with a silane primer to encourages bonding

Installs temporary composite veneers, which are removed at the next appointment

Wets the veneers and tests them for fit prior to cementation

Instructs the assistant to place a matrix strip between the teeth

Etches the enamel

Spreads a resin bonding agent over both etched enamel and the tooth side of the veneer

Applies a fine layer of the appropriate shade of resin bonding substance on the tooth side of the veneer

Instructs the assistant to light cure the site for about a minute

Finishes the site with suitable burrs and stones

Ceramic Restorations

All-ceramic restorations are for occlusal and multiple-surface restorations. Usually, the laboratory makes them with porcelain or castable glass, called Dicor. They can be constructed chairside, using CEREC computerized design, which is expensive but only takes one sitting. The dentist prepares the cavity and makes a final impression, an opposing arch alginate impression, and a bite registration. The dental ceramist makes the restoration. The dentist installs a temporary acrylic filling. Prior to insertion at the next appointment (or same day for CEREC), the dentist etches the porcelain and applies silanating agent for bonding. The dentist removes the temporary filing. The assistant cleans the tooth and positions matrix strips and wedges between proximal surface. The dentist etches the tooth, applies a bonding substance to the preparation, then dual-cure composite cement to both the preparation and the tooth side of the restoration. The dentist inserts the restoration and the assistant light cures it for about a minute on each surface. The dentist finishes it, tests the occlusion, and adjusts the restoration.

Cast-Gold Restorations

Cast-gold restorations include gold inlays, onlays, and bridges. All are made from gold alloys that have been melted and then cast and hardened into the needed shape. Gold alloys are readily melted, very strong to resist eating forces and edge fractures, non-corrosive, non-irritating, and non-allergenic. For gold inlays, the majority of the restoration is located within a tapered cavity in the tooth; these are appropriate for all cavity classes. Cast-gold onlays or crowns reach over the cusps of back teeth to ensure against fracture during mastication. Cast-gold crowns generally cover either three-quarters or the entire crown of the tooth. A three-quarter crown usually leaves the facial facet untouched for aesthetics. Cast-gold restorations always require two sittings: The first to prepare the tooth and take impressions before manufacture of the restoration in the laboratory (a temporary filling is inserted); and the second to fit and cement the restoration in place.

Cast-Gold Inlay Restorations

The dental assistant assists the dentist throughout the following procedures, and in some states is permitted to seat the retraction cord, make the final impression, and/or temporary filling. The dental team:
Uses alginate to make an impression of the opposing teeth that will abut the finished inlay

Fits the bite registration onto an articulator, incorporating the opposing model impression, if possible

Applies topical anesthetic

Injects local anesthetic

Isolates the site with cotton rolls

Removes the rubber dam (if any)

Retracts the gingival

Prepares the cavity with smooth, slightly tapered walls for later insertion of the inlay

Uses hemostatic agents to stop bleeding

Removes the cord

Dries the cavity preparation is dried

Takes an impression using agar hydrocolloid, polyether or polyvinylsiloxane

Temporizes the cavity preparation with a temporary filling of ZOE (zinc oxide and eugenol) or plastic

The procedure for the cementation appointment for cast-gold inlays is as follows: Apply anesthetics

Isolate the site with cotton rolls

Carefully remove the temporary with a spoon evacuator or burr, cotton pellets, and the air-water syringe

Seat the inlay with a wooden Coonley peg, orangewood stick, or other seating device

Check where the inlay contacts proximal surfaces of adjoining teeth and the cervical areas; make necessary adjustments

Tell the patient to bite down on articulating paper

Look for marks indicating hyperocclusion or too high an inlay; grind down, if any

Polish the final form with abrasives, externally on the tooth ,and then on the dental lathe

Disinfect the form
Wash, dry, and isolate the tooth for cementation

Pretreat the preparation with cavity varnish if using zinc phosphate cement; non-irritating polycarboxylate and glass ionomer cements is preferable

Blend the cement and layer it onto the prepared tooth surfaces

Position the inlay and seat it with finger pressure

Place a bite device over the inlay and instruct the patient to bite down until cement is set

Check and finish margins

Cast-Gold Crown

Teeth for which cast-gold crowns are fabricated have more area removed than those receiving inlays. Prepare them with a high-speed handpiece and tapered fissure burrs or diamond stones. For full crowns, grind the complete occlusal surface to a clearance of three thicknesses of occlusal wax (28 gauge sheets of wax). Three-quarter crowns leave the facial aspect intact. Temporary crowns for posterior teeth may employ either the:

Aluminum shell crown method, which uses stock aluminum shell crowns adjusted and temporarily cemented

Vacuum adaptation method for cast-gold crowns

Make a plaster model from an alginate impression

Make a plastic mold using a vacuum former with heating element (similar to making an acrylic resin custom tray)

Fill the appropriate part of the mold with self-curing acrylics

Place this over the prepared tooth while the patient bites down during hardening

Remove the mold and separate it from the acrylic

Polish

Seat with temporary cement

Sutures

Sutures are surgical seams for closing wounds. Sutures support healing, and reduce contamination with pathogens and food debris. The dental assistant helps the dentist insert sutures. Some states permit assistants to remove sutures. Here are the types of dental sutures, from most common to least common:

Simple suture, which is threaded through two skin areas and tied with a surgeon's knot

Continuous simple suture, which is a chain of sutures tied at either end with surgeon's knots, used for multiple extractions

Sling suture for interproximal areas, a threaded through the facial surface of the gum, enfolded around the lingual aspect of the tooth, put through the facial tissue on the other side of the tooth, wrapped back around the lingual side, and then the ends are tied

Continuous sling variant for a large opening, where the suture thread is wrapped onto the next tooth, instead of back around

Mattress sutures begin and end on the same aspect, e.g., the facial side, and the stitching is either horizontal or vertical

Suture Removal

Remove sutures when healing is indicated, usually between 5 and 7 days after insertion.

Set up a standard cart

Review the patient's chart

Debride the site using air and warm water spray, a cotton-tip applicator with water or dilute hydrogen peroxide, or moist cotton gauze

Inspect the suture site for location and number of sutures, the suture types and patterns, and healing of tissues in the region

For large areas with multiple extractions, healed areas look slightly red, with evidence of granulation tissue

If there was no periodontal dressing, there should be no infection

If periodontal dressing was performed, then a milky film should be in its place

For smaller areas where there was no periodontal dressing, the region should look fairly healed, with dark pink granulation tissue and no evidence of inflammation

Any wounds that are red, tender or bleeding are either infected, irritated or insufficiently healed

Confer with the dentist before suture removal

Use aseptic technique for all suture removal. You may only perform suture removal if the procedure is covered in your state under dental assistants' expanded functions. Otherwise, the dentist removes sutures. Do not disrupt the healing process; if you are unsure, consult the dentist before attempting removal. Control hemorrhaging by applying pressure with a gauze sponge. Do not cut knots. Do not pull exposed sutures and knots through the patient's tissue. For removal of simple or continuous simple sutures, gently lift the suture away from the tissues using a cotton plier. Cut the thread below the knot with a suture scissors near the tissue. Catch the knot in the pliers and pull it out. Place the suture on a gauze sponge for counting at the end of the procedure. Cut and remove each suture in a series of continuous simple sutures individually.

As with all other types of suture removal, sling removal is performed by the dentist or delegated to the expanded-function dental assistant if the state in which they practice permits it. Using aseptic techniques, the sling suture is severed in two places and loosened on both sides of the tooth with cotton pliers. The knot is pulled up and cut close to the tissue. The thread on the other side of the tooth is lifted with the pliers and cut. Each thread is taken out with the cotton pliers by drawing it toward the wrapped side. For example, a sling suture entered from the facial side and wrapped around the lingual side is pulled toward the latter during

- 47 -

removal. Sutures are placed on a gauze sponge for counting.

As with all other types of suture removal, mattress suture removal is performed by the dentist or delegated to the expanded-function dental assistant if the state in which they practice permits it. Horizontal mattress sutures are placed by horizontal stitching through one surface, followed by the same on the other aspect, and tying. Vertical mattress sutures have vertical stitching on each surface. Nevertheless, suture removal is similar for both. Lift the knot with cotton pliers. Sever the suture below the knot near the tissue. Make another cut close to the tissue on the other surface. Remove the suture by holding the knot with the cotton pliers and pulling up. Place the spent suture on the gauze sponge for later counting.

Enamel Sealants

Enamel sealants are hard resins spread over occlusal surfaces of children's premolars or molars with no decay. Sealants bind to the pits and fissures on the occlusal surface to lock out possible decay for five to seven years. Both deciduous and permanent, including newly erupted teeth, can be sealed. Sealants are especially indicated for patients with many other occlusal caries or deep fissures. Fluoridate the teeth in conjunction with sealing. Enamel sealants are inappropriate for teeth that are:

Decay-free for at least four years
Shallowly grooved, easy to clean, and decay-resistant

Well blended with pits and fissures

Already decayed

Restored
Resins enamel sealants are dilute concentrations of BIS-GMA dental composites or glass ionomers. They may be chemically cured two-paste systems or one-component light cured ones, and they may contain

fluoride. Perform pre-etching and conditioning before application with phosphoric acid because the enamel binding is mechanical.
Enamel sealing is performed by the dental assistant with expanded functions.

Polish the occlusal surface to be sealed with flour of pumice or prophy paste without fluoride. Use a rubber cup. Rinse and dry the area. Isolate it with a dental dam or cotton rolls. Dab acid etchant/conditioner (phosphoric acid solution) over the occlusal surface into the pits and fissures to the upper two-thirds of the cusp, until the area looks chalky and white. Rinse the tooth. Evacuate the mouth. Isolate tooth again with cotton rolls. Prepare sealant according to the manufacturer's suggested procedure. Place sealant into pits and fissures. Allow it to set (if self-curing) or light-cure it. Hold the curing light at the occlusal surface from 2 mm distance and expose it for up to one minute. Test the hardness and smoothness of the sealant with an explorer. Seal unsealed areas again, if necessary. After setting, rinse or wipe the tooth surface. Remove isolation materials. Check occlusion with articulating paper. Gently finish. Apply fluoride.

Bleaching

Non-vital bleaching means lightening endodontically treated (usually root canal) or non-vital teeth. The dentist bleaches teeth with assistance. Apply protective gel to soft tissues. Place a dental dam and a ligature of waxed dental floss around the indicated tooth or teeth. The dentist removes the crown restoration and debris and may scrub the open crown. The dentist applies a 2 to 3 mm layer of base cement, light-cured resin ionomer, or bonded composite to the top of the root canal to ensure bleach does not enter the root. There are two options for the actual non-vital bleaching:
Gel bleaching in the office, which entails filling the chamber with bleaching gel for 30 minutes, with bleach changes every 10 minutes (and possibly heat application),

followed by cotton roll isolation and placement of a temporary crown. Requires 3 appointments spaced 3 to7 days apart. Walking bleaching, this is placement of a viscous paste of hydrogen peroxide and/or sodium perborate into the crown and covering it with temporary cement. Requires 3 appointments, space 2 to 5 days apart.

Finally, remove the temporary filling and install the permanent filling. Veneers may be indicated.

Teeth can be bleached to remove both extrinsic stains from habits like coffee-drinking, and intrinsic stains from root canals, tetracycline use, damage, or fluorosis. Use sodium perborate, hydrogen peroxide, or carbamide peroxide. In-office bleaching of vital teeth is performed by the dentist with assistance. Smear protective gel on adjacent tissues. Isolate the area with a dental dam and a ligature of waxed floss surrounding each tooth. Polish teeth crowns with pumice or prophy gel. Mix bleaching materials according to the manufacturer's directions until thick. Apply directly onto the facial and lingual facades of the teeth or in a tray. Some materials require use of heat or light, or reapplication of fresh gel every 10 minutes. After bleaching, rinse. Remove the dam and ligatures. Polish teeth with a resin polishing cup or prophy paste containing fluoride. Home bleaching involves taking an alginate impression, from which a cast and custom trays are made. The patient uses the trays at home with a bleaching kit, as directed.

Cavity Liners, Cavity Varnish and Cement Bases

These procedures are executed by the dentist or the expanded-function dental assistant. Cavity liners include calcium hydroxide, glass ionomer or zinc oxide eugenol. Prepare as directed. Apply to the clean and dry cavity preparation. Place liner only into the deepest part of the preparation, using a ball attachment. Liners are either self-curing or light-cured for 10 to 20 seconds.

Cavity varnish seals dentin tubules. Painted a thin layer over all exposed dentin with a cotton ball or pellet and sterile cotton pliers. Apply a second coat. Avoid contaminating the varnish.

Cement bases are applied to the cleaned cavity preparation after a cavity liner and/or varnish. Mix the cement base materials as directed to a thick texture. Place onto the floor of the cavity preparation using a plastic filling instrument. Allow room for the restorative material.

Chairside Dental Materials

Impression Trays

Impression trays document tooth areas. They are for diagnosis, making temporary dental crowns, or developing an indirect casting. Commercially-available stock or preformed trays are used for preliminary and final impressions and temporary needs. They are sold in various sizes and materials, including metal, Styrofoam, and tough plastic. Impression trays can cover the full arch, a half arch (quadrant tray), or just the front teeth (section tray). Some are perforated, so the impression material bonds with the tray. Customized trays specially made for an individual are made of lightweight resins, either light-cured, acrylic or thermoplastic. They are used for final impressions, making temporary restorations, or vital bleaching (external surface teeth whitening).

Preliminary Impressions

An impression is a negative copy of teeth and adjacent structures. Preliminary impressions are diagnostic models for preparation of orthodontic and dental appliances, and provisional dental crowns. Impressions record tooth condition prior to and after treatment, especially for custom impressions. Preliminary impressions are created by the dentist or assistant (if legally allowed by the state) from alginate, a hydrocolloid comprised of potassium alginate and other compounds. Alginate is sold as a powder, to which the assistant adds an equal amount of water. The material first goes through a sol or solution phase that is liquid or semi-liquid. It proceeds to a gel or semisolid phase. Use 2 or 3 scoops of powder and equal measures of water for mandibular or maxillary impressions. Working time is 2 minutes for normal set and 1¼ minutes for fast set.

Normal and fast sets have setting times of 4½ and 1 to 2 minutes, respectively.

Alginate has short working and setting times. The dentist or assistant should be positioned so that insertion is quick and controlled. The impression tray containing the alginate mixture is turned a bit initially, so the team can place a corner of it into the patient's mouth. Retract the patient's cheek out of the way. Slide the tray into the mouth. Center it over the teeth. Seat the back part of the tray before the front part, to prevent alginate flowing into the mouth and throat. Push the tray into place very gently. Pull the patient's lips out around the tray. Hold securely in place until the alginate sets.

Diagnostic Casts

A diagnostic cast is a positive mock-up of the teeth and surrounding structures created by filling in the impression with model plaster or dental stone. Model plaster is the weaker material and is more easily trimmed. It is related to plaster of Paris. Dental stone is more robust and is the material of choice for retainers and custom trays. Both model plaster and dental stone contain gypsum, but a higher proportion of water is added to set model plaster than dental stone, or its stronger relative, high-strength stone. Setting time is affected by the type of gypsum, the water-powder ratio, length and speed of mixing, water temperature, and ambient humidity. Reduce setting time with a lower water-powder ratio, long or intense mixing, water temperature above room temperature, or on a humid day. Use the double-pour, box-and-pour, or inverted-pour methods. Trim and finish using a model trimmer. The end-product has two portions: An anatomic part showing the teeth, mucosa and muscle attachments (2/3), and an art portion or base (1/3).

Final Impressions

Final impressions provide more precise definition of the teeth and surrounding

- 50 -

structures of interest than preliminary impressions. Occasionally, alginate is used for final impressions, but more often elastomeric impression materials are chosen. Two compounds are mixed together to create the final elastomeric material: A base and a catalyst. The various choices are defined by their viscosity or capacity to flow. Light, regular and heavy body materials are increasing thick. Heavy body is the most commonly used. There are four types of final impression materials available: Polysulfide, polyether, condensation silicone, and addition silicone. In terms of stiffness and stability, the best choice is addition stone, followed by polyether.

Making final impressions is a two-person job. The assistant mixes. The dentist takes the impression.

Mixing time is a minute or less for all final impression materials. Setting time averages 6 minutes for all, except polysulfide, which takes 10 to 20 minutes to set. If the base and catalyst come as two pastes, they are mixed either by swirling them together and smoothing them with a spatula, or by using an automix system. The automix system consists of extruder units with cartridges of the base and catalyst, which are mixed when a trigger is squeezed. Segregate the tooth for which the impression is taken by a retraction system. Rinse and dry. Insert a recently-mixed light-body impression material is into the sulcus, around the tooth, and into adjacent areas. Mix the heavy-body material and place it into the impression tray. Load it in place over the light-body material. After setting, remove the impression. Examine and disinfect it. Placed in into a labeled precaution bag for transport to the laboratory.

Gingival retraction uses a cord to briefly push the gingival tissue away from a tooth and broaden the sulcus. Gingival retraction cords isolate a tooth for the final impression. Dry the tooth. Separate the quadrant with cotton rolls. Loop the retraction cord and slide it over the tooth. Push it into the sulcus in a clockwise motion with a cord-packing device. The end of the cord should end up on the facial side, where it remains sticking out, you may place it into the sulcus. After several minutes, remove the retraction cord counterclockwise with cotton pliers. Dry the area and apply new cotton rolls. Procure the impression quickly. Sometimes, chemical retraction is used in conjunction with these procedures by initial use of a topical hemostatic solution, aluminum salt astringents, or epinephrine (an astringent and vasoconstrictor). Retraction can also be performed with a surgical knife or electric cauterizer.

Occlusal Registrations

Occlusal or bite registrations are impressions that document the centric relationship between a patient's maxillary and mandibular arches. The centric relationship is the position of optimally stable connection between occlusal surfaces of the two arches when the mouth is closed. Bite registrations are made of wax or paste, both of which do not flow easily. If wax is used, heat it for softening. Place wax directly onto the occlusal surfaces. The patient bites down lightly into the wax until it cools. Remove the registration and store it Pastes set quickly, are odorless and tasteless, and conform easily to biting. Pastes have two cartridges or parts that are mixed. Spread right over the teeth or put in a gauze tray, and then the patient bites down for the impression.

Biting Forces

Anything that exerts a push or pull on an object is a force. The object resists the force, causing stress. Significant stress causes a strain or alteration in the object. Three forms of stress and strain can occur:

Tensile force, or outward stretching and pulling, potentially causing elongation. Elastic bands used in orthodontics can cause tensile stress and strain.

Compressive force or pushing together, which occurs during chewing or biting.

Shearing or portions sliding across one another from side to side, such as when people grind their teeth (bruxism). It is important to select dental materials that can withstand tensile and compressive forces, properties known as ductility and malleability, respectively.

All of these types of stress and strain apply to dentistry; consider them when selecting dental materials, because biting forces are significant. People bite down on molars with forces in the range of 130 to 170 pounds, and about a quarter of that is on incisors.

Acidity

The parameter pH is a measurement of the relative acidity, neutrality or alkalinity of a solution or environment. It is quantified on a scale from 0 to 14. Low numbers indicate acidic environments. pH 7.0 is neutral. High numbers indicate alkalinity. Normally, the oral cavity is maintained at relative neutrality by saliva. However, sugary and acidic foods and bacteria cause ongoing fluctuations in pH. Select dental materials to withstand these fluctuations. Some dental materials themselves are acidic and potentially damaging to gum tissues or pulp. If used, acidic materials must be set up and inserted cautiously.

Thermal Properties

The important thermal properties of a potential dental material are its thermal conductivity and its thermal expansion. Thermal conductivity refers to the facility to convey heat. Materials with lower thermal conductivity are preferred usually particularly if they are near the dental pulp. Thermal expansion refers to the rate of expansion and contraction when exposed to temperature variations. It is important to select a material that has thermal expansion rates similar to that of tooth structure.

Thermal expansion can cause dimensional changes in the dental material, particularly during the setting process. This can result in a phenomenon called microleakage in which debris and saliva leak into the area between the tooth and restorative material. Later, tooth sensitivity or caries can result.

Retention

Retention is the act of keeping or holding something in place. In dentistry, retention is achieved by either mechanical or chemical means. Dental materials are held in place by mechanical retention by slanting the cavity walls inward, abrading the tooth surface with an etchant, or by furrowing the cavity walls. Chemical retention is achieved by some sort of chemical reaction between the dental material and the tooth surface. It is often used for insertion of gold inlays or crowns, which must be indirectly retained through use of cements or bonding agents.

Other Dental Material Properties

Some important properties of dental materials to consider before selection include:
Adhesion - the ability of dissimilar materials to stick together, either chemically or physically

Elasticity - the capacity to undergo distortion and return to the original conformation, such as rubber bands within their elastic limit

Flow - gradual continual shape change under force, such as compression-associated amalgam changes

Hardness - relative ability to resist scratching or denting

Solubility - capacity to dissolve in fluid; extremely soluble materials are undesirable if in contact with saliva

Viscosity - thickness or facility of a liquid to flow

Wettability - the capacity of a liquid (the dental material) to flow over and sink into another (the tooth)

Corrosiveness - the ability to react with food or saliva causing pitting, coarseness or tarnishing, with metal-containing materials

Galvanism - electric shock caused by reaction between dissimilar metals and carried by saliva

Dental Cements

Dental cements are agents that bond other dental materials, like restorations to the teeth. Cements come in various forms that generally require mixing and preparation before use. The cements are hardened either by chemical self-curing or light curing with a special blue light. Cements are defined as temporary, intermediate, or permanent, depending on their expected duration. There are also thin liners that are used to seal and protect the pulp or wall and floor of the cavity. Bases are relatively strong dental cements that are thickly spread in a layer between the tooth and restoration for pulp protection. Besides restorations, cements are also utilized as luting or bonding agents to apply orthodontic bands, bridges, or inlays to the teeth.

Most dental cements are permanent, including zinc phosphate, reinforced zinc oxide eugenol, polycarboxylate, glass ionomer, resin cement, resin-reinforced glass ionomer, and compomers. The cements that are used for permanent cementation of orthodontic bands and brackets are zinc phosphate, polycarboxylate, glass ionomer and resin cement, all of which are bases and used to cement crowns, inlays, onlays and bridges. Glass ionomer is also utilized to seal root canals and for restorations. Reinforced zinc oxide eugenol is not used for orthodontic work. Resin cement is employed for cementation of enzootic posts, ceramic or composite inlays and onlays, and resin-bonded bridges. Compomers are resins altered with polyacid. Resin-reinforced glass ionomer is used for metallic or porcelain-fused metallic restorations. Zinc oxide eugenol is used only for temporary cementation of crowns, inlays, onlays and bridges, as a root canal sealant, or as a periodontal dressing after surgery. Varnish and calcium hydroxide are examples of liners.

Zinc Phosphate Cements

Zinc oxide cement preparations are composed of two parts that are mixed together. The first is a powder made of zinc oxide, and a small quantity of magnesium oxide, and tints of white, yellow or gray. The second part is a buffered phosphoric acid solution. When the two are combined, a heat-liberating or exothermic reaction occurs, which must be dampened during preparation by using a cooled glass slab and spatula. The mixture hardens within about 5 minutes and is very strong. The mechanism of bonding is mechanical interlocking. The desired consistency depends on the use; it should be creamy in texture for luting and similar to thick putty for use as a base.

The dental or orthodontic assistant mixes the zinc phosphate cement on a clean, cooled glass slab. The powder portion is spread, flattened, and divided with a stainless steel cement spatula on one end of the slab.. The liquid portion is dispensed with the dropper bottle unto the other end. The flat side of the spatula is used to integrate a portion of the powder into the liquid for about 15 seconds. The mixture is spread over a larger area of the slab and slowly more powder is mixed in with the spatula until the desired thickness is achieved. The mass is formed into a ball and transferred to the dentist on the slab under the person's chin. The assistant also transfers a plastic filling instrument to the dentist. The slab and spatula are wiped with moistened gauze, soaked in water or bicarbonate,, and then sterilized or disinfected.

Zinc Oxide Eugenol Cements

Zinc oxide eugenol (ZOE) cement comes in two types. The traditional type I preparation consists of a powder containing zinc oxide, zinc acetate, resin, and an accelerator, which are mixed with the liquid eugenol. ZOE is used only for temporary cementation or for post-surgical periodontal dressing because of its soothing properties. The variant type II preparation is reinforced with alumina and other resins and alumina in the powder and ethoxybenzoic acid in the eugenol, and it is useful for up to a year as an Intermediate Restorative Material (IRM). Zinc oxide eugenol is very soluble and of neutral pH. When reinforced, ZOE is also strong. ZOE is incompatible with acrylic or composite restorations. Mixing is done on either a paper pad or glass slab, using a stainless steel cement spatula. Eugenol disintegrates rubber, so it should not meet the bulb. ZOE preparations are not used for orthodontic procedures.

For powder/liquid systems:
The dental assistant dispenses the powder onto the mixing pad (paper or glass), followed by the liquid. The two should be placed near but not on top of each other. Mix the two with the cement spatula, using the flat part of the instrument and uniform pressure. Consolidate the mixture into a mass to check for consistency, which should be creamy for luting applications, and similar to putty if needed as an insulating base or intermediate restorative material. Transfer the material to the dentist under the individual's chin, using a plastic filling instrument. Wipe off both the spatula and plastic filling instrument after use. If a paper pad was used, remove the top paper. If a glass slab was used, clean it with alcohol or orange solvent.

The dental assistant mixes and distributes pastes. If state law allows, the assistant can place pastes. If the law does not allow this extended responsibility, the assistant aids the dentist in placement of these preparations.

Two-paste systems are used for temporary bonding. They consist of an accelerator and a base. Each paste is spread parallel to the other along a paper pad. A cement spatula is used to mix the two until they have a creamy texture, suitable for luting. This process is very fast (about 15 minutes), as is the setting time (5 minutes or less). The material is put in place with the plastic filling instrument. The cement spatula is wiped off with a gauze sponge.

Polycarboxylate Cements

Polycarboxylate cements are mainly used for permanent cementation of orthodontic bands and brackets. Polycarboxylate cements consist of two portions, which are mixed. The first is a powder, containing primarily zinc oxide, with smaller amounts of magnesium oxide and stannous fluoride. The second is a thick liquid made of polycyclic acid copolymer in water. Polycarboxylate cements adhere chemically to the teeth and mechanically to the restoration. They are relatively strong and non-irritating to the pulp. The chemical reaction does not release heat. These cements must be prepared and used quickly, as they have a mixing time of a minute or less and operational time of approximately three minutes, after which unutilized cement should be discarded when it appears dull or sinewy.

The dental assistant mixes cement. Place powder on one side of a paper pad or glass slab and drops of the liquid on the other. Manufacturer's directions should indicate the ratio of drops to scoops of powder. The relative amount of water is less if a base consistency is desired, or if the preparation is to be used for bonding. The powder is quickly incorporated into the liquid with some pressure for wetting. The mixture should have a glossy texture. For luting purposes, it should adhere to the spatula somewhat if raised an inch. It should be stickier for use as a base. The mixture should be applied within about 3 minutes, before it develops a dull and/or sinewy appearance.

- 54 -

The spatula is wiped off with wet gauze, or bathed in 10% NaOH, if the cement has dried. Dispose of the paper pad.

Glass Ionomer Cements

There are five types of glass ionomer cements:

Type I is conventional, viscous, or condensable. It has fine grains and chemically binds to the tooth. Use it for orthodontic bonding and closing fissures and pits.

Type II is conventional modified with resin by the addition of HEMA. It is coarser and is for restorations.

Type III is dual-cured hybrid for luting.

Type IV is tri-cured glass for opaque structures. It releases less fluoride than conventional glass ionomers.

Type V is any metal reinforced admixture containing glass ionomers; it is used with silver or amalgam restorations for crown or core buildups.

Unless reinforced, these cements come as a silicate glass powder containing calcium, fluoride and aluminum, and an aqueous suspension of polycyclic acid. Glass ionomer cements are quite strong. They bond both chemically and mechanically to the teeth, discharge fluoride, and are relatively non-irritating. While the setting and working times are short, about 1 and 2 minutes respectively, these cements do not set completely for about a day. Resin-reinforced glass ionomer cements are stronger, less water-soluble, and more adherent.

The dental assistant first rinses and evacuates the patient's mouth . Dispense the powder and then the liquid portions onto a paper pad or cool glass stab. Immediately recap the liquid to avoid evaporation. Work quickly. Move a portion of the powder into the liquid with a flexible stainless steel spatula. Mix and incorporate the remaining powder until the proper consistency is achieved. If the cement is for luting orthodontic work, the texture should be creamy and glossy. If it is a base, then the consistency should be stickier. Transfer the mixture to the dentist under the patient's chin along with the plastic filling instrument. Cleanup involves wiping off the instruments with a moistened gauze and disposal of the top paper. If glass ionomer capsules are used instead, the seal between the powder and liquid sides is broken in an activator and the tablets are mixed for about 10 seconds on an amalgamator. Place the capsule in a dispenser and transfer it to the dentist for application. Discard the remainder and disinfect your equipment.

Calcium Hydroxide Cements

Calcium hydroxide cements are placed in thin layers to protect the pulp by gently chafing the pulp enough to encourage secondary dentin formation. They are also used as liners under restorations. Calcium hydroxide cements are not very strong. Their formulations contain other chemicals, in addition to the calcium hydroxide, and may be either self-curing or light-curing. The most common system consists of two pastes, one of which is the base, and the other the catalyst for the reaction. With a two-paste system, equivalent small quantities of base and catalyst are dispensed onto a paper pad. The two are blended quickly (up to 15 seconds), using a small ball-ended instrument or explorer and a circular motion, until a consistent color is achieved. The assistant transfers the on the pad to the dentist under the patient's chin. The duration before setting can be from 2 to 7 minutes, depending on the preparation. The assistant wipes the instrument between applications and afterwards discards the paper pad.

Cavity Varnish

Cavity varnishes close up dentin tubules before an amalgam restoration. They are applied in a thin layer to the dentin. All preparations contain some type of resin. Place universal varnishes under any restoration materials. Varnishes that include organic solvents are called copal varnishes, which are only appropriate under metal fillings. Varnishes are one of the weakest types of restorative materials, but they are impenetrable to oral fluids and are useful against microleakage or infiltration of cement acids into the dentin. The dental assistant prepares cavity varnishes. Your state may allow you to apply varnish, or may stipulate the dentist does. The patient's mouth should be clean and dry. Apply two coats of varnish using two small cotton pellets and two cotton pliers. While holding it in the pliers, moisten the first pellet with the varnish. Recap the varnish to avoid evaporation. Dab away extra varnish with gauze. Coat the desired surface using the cotton pellet. After drying, repeat the procedure with the second pellet and pliers. Discard pellets. Wash the pliers with solvent.

Resin Cement

Resin cements are made up of bisphenol A-glycidyl methacrylate (BIS-GMA) or dimethacrylate resins, in combination with low-viscosity monomers, and sometimes fluoride. The cements do not bond directly to metal or ceramics. Instead, an etchant must first be applied to the tooth surface, or a silane coupling agent must be used to achieve mechanical or chemical bonding, respectively. Resin cements have a variety of applications. The curing method is related to the application. Self-curing or chemical-cured cements, which have an initiator and activator that are mixed, are used with metal restoration materials or endodontic posts. Orthodontic brackets and porcelain/resin restorations or veneers indicate use of light cured materials, which are supplied in syringes. There are also dual-cured materials that come in two parts, which are mixed, applied, and light-cured. There are polyacid-modified compomer cements with similar properties.

Clean the tooth surface beforehand. Segregate the site with cotton rolls. The dental assistant prepares the etchant applicator and holds it on the tooth surface, per manufacturer's specifications, up to 30 seconds. The etchant may be transferred to and applied by the dentist. With the dual-curing method of resin cement placement, the tooth is then dried and the adhesive applied. The assistant quickly mixes resin components, initiator and activator on a paper pad with a stainless steel spatula to a uniform, creamy consistency. The assistant transfers the pad near to the patient, along with the plastic filling instrument. The placement is performed by the dentist. The assistant sets up the curing light. Actual curing or hardening may be done by the dentist or assistant, using the curing light and a protective shield or glasses when the light is on. Gauze sponges are used for cleanup and disposables are thrown out.

Bonding Agents

Bonding agents are materials that adhere restoration materials to either dentin or enamel. They are also referred to as adhesives or bonding resins. The main constituents of bonding agents are low-viscosity resins and sometimes fillers, enhancers, or fluoride. Most preparations are light-cured or dual-cured. In order for bonding to occur, surface alteration or scoring needs is performed before the bonding agent can penetrate the surface and form a mechanical bond. For enamel bonding, the first step is acid etching using phosphoric acid. Bonding to the more-sensitive, organic and water-filled dentin is achieved by initially slashing the dentin with a burr, and then using an etchant to eliminate the resulting smear layer.

Bonding systems consist of the acid etchant, primer or conditioner, and the adhesive or bonding agent. The dental assistant is responsible for preparation and transfer of materials and maintenance of a dry and clean area. If the procedure is in close contact with the pulp, the first step is placement of lining cement, such as calcium hydroxide. The etchant is then applied to the enamel and then the dentin. Manufacturer's instructions indicate the correct application time. The tooth is rinsed. A brush or disposable applicator is used to apply a primer, which moistens the dentin, and seeps into the tubules. The bonding agent is then placed and solidified, using a curing light. Disposable tips or brushes are thrown away.

Alginate Impression Material

Alginate is a general term for irreversible hydrocolloid impression materials. These materials make impressions for diagnostic casts and study models. Their main application in orthodontic work is as negative models for preparation of casts that can be used to formulate orthodontic appliances. Hydrocolloid impressions are also taken to make opposite models for prosthetics, temporary restorations, bleach trays, custom trays, and mouth guards. The main ingredient is marine-derived potassium alginate. It is soluble in water, forming a thick liquid or sol. When calcium sulfate is added, solidification (a gel) occurs. Hydrocolloid impression materials also contain trisodium phosphate, which slows down setting time, fillers like diatomaceous earth or zinc oxide for strength, and potassium titanium fluoride. Alginate is extensively used because it is easy, cheap, and comfortable to use, it sets quickly, and little equipment is needed. Its elastic properties make it ideal for making impressions where there are recessed areas, and both tissue and teeth imprints can be taken. The major disadvantage is the possibility of some inaccuracy in the impression, due to changes in water content. Heat, dryness, or contact with air can result in syneresis or shrinkage of the material. Water gain can result in imbibition or an enlargement of the measurements of the impression. Tissue areas being imprinted may be distorted because of the thickness of the material. Other impression materials, such as elastomer, are more accurate.

Irreversible hydrocolloid impression materials or alginate may come packaged in: Hermetic plastic containers, with foil or plastic bags inside, containing the powder and measuring tools for water

Mixtures in sealed bags
Mixtures used with a dispensing unit

Store irreversible hydrocolloid impression materials in areas where they will not be exposed to moisture or excessive heat. Shelf life is about one year. The method of mixing the powder and water is specified by the manufacturer. In general the ratio between the two is 1:1, but two scoops of powder and two portions of water are used for mandibular impressions, while three of each is required for maxillary impressions. If too little water is added, the mixture will be too thick, and vice versa.

The period between which the water is added to the powder and the total setting of the mixture is the gelatin time. This includes approximately one minute of working time for Type II regular-set alginate and less for fast-set Type I. Setting time occurs after that, in approximately 1 to 2 minutes for Type I or 2 to 4½ minutes for Type II, if the impression is taken at normal room temperature, about 70°F. Both working and setting times are shortened at higher temperatures and lengthened at lower temperatures, for example, with use of cool water. In general, Type I is useful for children or people who tend to gag, whereas the slower setting Type II is convenient for more difficult insertions or in situations where there is only one operator.

Dispensing units using premixed units require only dispensing tips. The mixture is distributed directly into the tray. When mixing of the powder and water, use flexible rubber bowls and throwaway spatulas (generally two-sided for mixing of alginate or plaster). The bowl is sterilized or sanitized afterwards. There are also disposable spatulas and bowls with markings for water

- 57 -

measurement. There are metal impression trays that must be sterilized after use and disposable plastic trays. Most have perforations to allow material through and keep it in place. There are also unperforated rim lock trays with rims to hold the impression material in place. Trays come in various sizes and should be selected so they fit the person's mouth, with room for 2 mm of the hydrocolloid. They should also reach several millimeters posterior to the molar area; if they do not, they can be extended using wax strips (beading).

If legally allowed by the state, the dental assistant can take an alginate impression. The patient should be sitting up, with mouth is rinsed and evacuated. Test the impression trays for size. If the selected tray does not extend beyond the molars, add wax beading to the borders. Prepare the mandibular model first. Add two measurements of room temperature water to one flexible mixing bowl, followed by two scoops of water in another bowl. Fluff the powder needs beforehand. Add the powder to the water and mix with the spatula, first by stirring, and then by applying pressure with the smooth side of the spatula on the side of the basin. Mixing time should be about 30 to 45 seconds for fast set, or 60 seconds for regular set preparations. A creamy, uniform consistency is desired. Put the preparation in the impression tray, starting from the lingual sides. The flat edge (and sometimes a moist, gloved hand) consolidates the material. Maxillary impressions, which have a greater tendency to cause choking, are prepared similarly later, except that 3 measurements of water and 3 scoops of powder are used.

In some states, the dental assistant is legally allowed to take alginate impressions. Prepare the alginate. The operator faces the patient to take the mandibular impression. Draw the patient's right cheek back slightly. Spread alginate over the occlusal surfaces. Turn the impression tray over with the alginate facing the teeth. Insert the tray through the lips one side at a time, until it is centered above the teeth. Settle the back portion of the tray into the teeth first. Instruct the patient to lift and move his/her tongue to insure the alveolar process is part of the imprint. The operator pulls out the patient's lip and concludes by placing the tray down, while pushing toward the back. Hold the tray in place with a finger on each side, toward the back, with the patient's lip around the tray near the handle. The alginate is set when it is stiff and fixed. The maxillary impression tray is loaded similarly, except that the tray faces upward and a little of the alginate in the tray needs to be removed from the palate region before insertion.

Begin removal by using the fingers of one hand to break the seal between the tissues of the lips and the cheek and the tray. shield the opposite arch with your opposite hand. Abruptly remove the tray with a snapping motion, pulling up for the maxillary impression and down for the mandibular. Turn the tray a bit sideways for removal. Evacuate surplus alginate from the mouth. Tissue off surplus alginate from the face. Ask the patient to rinse and spit. Examine the impression for accuracy. Rinse it with tap water and spray it with an approved surface disinfectant, such as an iodophor. Alginate impressions that are not poured into casts immediately (within 20 minutes) should be enclosed in a labeled, covered container until use. If the impression is wrapped first in a moist towel, it leads to water intake and distortion over time.

Accurate alginate impressions are centered over the central incisors, include all essential areas, and illustrate well-defined anatomic detail of both teeth and tissues. The teeth should not pierce through to the tray, caused by pushing the tray up or down too far. The imprint should not have tears, bubbles or empty spaces. It should encompass the vestibule regions and have a good peripheral or marginal roll Certain features should be evident. For the mandibular impression, these are retromolar area, the lingual frenum and the mylohyoid ridge region. For the maxillary impression, these are the tuberosities and the palate regions.

Agar Impression Material

Reversible hydrocolloid impression material, also known as agar-agar, is similar in makeup to alginate. The difference is that hydrocolloid setting is achieved through a chemical reaction. The material is transformed from a gel to sol state by boiling for 10 minutes in a hydrocolloid conditioner unit. It is maintained in a liquid state in a 150°F water bath until about 5 minutes before use, at which time it is moved to an 110°F water bath. Further cooling to convert the material back to a gel occurs in the mouth, using hoses connected to the dental unit. Reversible hydrocolloid materials are quite accurate, making them useful for final impressions and other applications requiring detail. The disadvantages of hydrocolloid include the expense of additional equipment, longer preparation and setting (10 minutes), and distortion over time if exposed to environmental changes.

Use a three-compartment hydrocolloid conditioning unit. The separate sections all contain clean water maintained at different temperatures. Looking toward the unit, from the left the partitions are the boiling bath (150°F, 66°C), the storage bath (usually 110°F, 45°C), and the conditioning bath (water-cooled tray). The impression material is provided in collapsible plastic tubes or syringes, which are shuttled between the three compartments after the appropriate time. If tubes are used, they are positioned upside down, with tips tightly in place in each compartment. Syringes have special holding cases for the cartridge. Time must either be set digitally or watched by the dental assistant, particularly the boiling time (10 minutes) and conditioning bath (5 minutes). The tray must be cool enough for insertion to avoid burning the patient's mouth. Otherwise, taking the hydrocolloid impression is similar to use of alginate, except that the setting time is longer, about 10 minutes.

Elastomeric Impression Materials

Elastomeric impression materials are more flexible than other types. This means they are less prone to tearing and distortion upon removal. They are also relatively impervious to temperature changes. There are three general types of elastomeric impression materials: Polysulfide, silicone, and polyether. Each type is prepared by mixing a catalyst or accelerator and a base material, engendering a process called polymerization. During the polymerization process, the material converts from a paste into a rubber-like, elastic mass. Elastomeric impression materials are mixed using either a mixing pad and spatula, or an extruder gun, to which cartridges of base and catalyst and a mixing tip are attached externally.

The pros and cons of elastomeric impression materials are:

Polysulfide - It comes as a two-paste system, with a base of thiodol polysulfide rubber and filler and a catalyst of lead peroxide. Material is stable after setting, very precise, and has a long shelf life. However, it has a sulfurous odor, stains, and long setting time (at least 10 minutes).

Silicone - It comes as two color-coded putties, a base of polysiloxane or polyvinyl siloxanes, and a catalyst. The putties are mixed and dispensed using an extruder gun. Silicone impression materials are highly accurate, stable, odorless, tasteless, and do not shrink or change measurements. They are relatively expensive.

Polyether - It comes as a color-coded two paste system. The pastes (base and catalyst) are spread in parallel on a paper pad and mixed with a spatula. Polyether systems are quite accurate and stable.

Polysulfide Impressions

Polysulfide impressions are taken by the dentist, supported by one or two assistants. The patient is sitting up. Rinse and evacuate the patient's mouth. Two different mixtures are prepared by separate individuals: One mixture for loading onto a syringe, and another for loading onto the impression tray. Parallel, non-touching lines of base and accelerator pastes are dispensed onto two paper pads. Each is mixed using a spatula, with the mixing of the syringe preparation initiated about a minute before that for the tray. Place the syringe preparation into an impression syringe that has an attached tip. Remove the cylinder by forcing it into the barrel, using the working end. Insert the plunger. Transfer the syringe to the dentist, who applies the material to the prepared tooth. Load the tray mixture into the impression tray with a spatula, smooth it out, and pass it to the dentist for insertion. Hold the tray in place for setting, a minimum of 6 minutes. Clean the spatula by pulling the material off, followed by sterilization. Discard the paper sheet and disposables.

Silicone Impressions

The dental assistant supports the dentist. The patient sits erect. Don vinyl gloves. Silicone impression materials come as two color-coded putties and scoops (base and catalyst), or a putty base and catalyst in liquid dropper form. Blend equal amounts and mold them into a homogenous patty. Load the patty into a stock tray with adhesive, within 30 seconds. Forge a dent where the affected teeth are to be placed. Place a plastic spacer sheet over the tray and place it in the patient's mouth. Remove the tray and spacer after about 3 minutes and allow the preliminary impression to set. Position a retraction cord over the desired tooth, in preparation for the final impression. Use an extruder gun because it mixes and dispenses a lighter body silicone preparation. Force some of the material through a mixing tip into the preliminary impression tray. Use an intraoral delivery tip to inject some material around the prepared tooth, after retraction cord removal. The dentist places and holds the tray in place a minimum of 3 minutes until set. Remove the impression, rinse, gently dry, and disinfect it.

Bite Registrations

Bite registrations are performed by the dental assistant under supervision, or by the dentist, aided by the assistant. Use either bite registration wax or polysiloxane. Sit the patient upright. Teach the patient how to bite in occlusion before the registration. If bite registration wax is used, determine the correct length, warm and soften it with water or a torch, and then place it on the mandibular occlusal edges. If polysiloxane is used, force the material through an extruder gun with disposable tip, right onto the occlusal surfaces. The assistant watches to ensure the patient bites with proper occlusion, as previously directed. The patient holds the occlusion for a minute or two, while the wax cools, or until the polysiloxane hardens. Remove the bite material. Disinfect and label the impression. Store it for later use.

Polyether Impressions

Spread the two pastes, containing the base and catalyst, in parallel lines onto a paper pad. Quickly mix them for 30 seconds or less, using a spatula. Put the paste into the impression tray and hand it to the dentist for the preliminary impression The dentist positions the tray and holds it about 3 minutes in the patient's mouth before removal. About 2 minutes into this process, the tray is moved around. For the final impression, the base, catalyst, and sometimes a consistency modifier (for thinning) are mixed and forced into the open end of an injection syringe. This material is put into the preliminary impression, and the tray is reintroduced into the patient's mouth. Hold it in the mouth about 4 minutes. Remove it abruptly with a snapping motion. Rinse, dry,

and disinfect the impression for 10 minutes
with 2% glutaraldehyde. Sometimes, only
final polyether impressions are made.

Laboratory Materials and Procedures

Gypsum Materials

Gypsum materials are used to make impressions for dental models. All gypsum products are made from mined hard rock, heated to remove water in a process known as calcinations, which changes the ratio of calcium sulfate to water from 1:2 to 2:1 (from calcium sulfate dihydrate to hemihydrates). The resultant material is pulverized and colored; the particle size and color are indicative of the type of gypsum product. Finely ground gypsum materials are denser, stronger, and require less water for wetting and setting. When water is added to the particles, they convert back to the dihydrate form, discharging heat in an exothermic reaction. Setting is virtually complete when the model is cool to the touch, although complete setting may take a day. The setting time is conversely related to the water temperature. The water-to-powder ratio is crucial, as it determines strength and fluidity ,and cannot be changed once setting has begun.

There are five types of gypsum dental products. Proceeding from Type I to Type V, the particles are finer, denser, stronger, and require less water for optimal setting.

Type	Main Use	Add water per 100 grams powder
Type I	Impression plaster for impressions	60 mL
Type II	Model or laboratory plaster for casts/models	50 mL
Type III	Laboratory stone	30 mL
Type IV	Die stone for strong or dyed models	24 mL
Type V	High-strength, high-expansion die stone	18 to 22 mL

Orthodontic stone is a combination of Type II laboratory plaster and Type III laboratory stone. Plaster is calcinated by an open kettle technique, making the particles very irregular and permeable. Die stone is processed by autoclaving with calcium chloride, making it denser and more uniform. Stone is alpha-hemihydrate. Plaster is beta-hemihydrate.

Pouring Alginate Impressions

The dental assistant makes the impression. Measure 50 ml of room temperature water into a flexible mixing bowl. Weigh 100 grams of plaster into another flexible bowl. Transfer the powder into the bowl with the water and let it dissolve. This makes a Type II model or laboratory plaster. Blend the particles with a metal spatula for about a minute. Press and rotate the bowl on a vibrator platform for several minutes, set at low to medium speed. This process introduces air bubbles that form to the top of the mixture. The desired consistency is creamy and smooth, but thick enough to remain in position.

The dental assistant makes the study model. Mix the plaster and pour it into the alginate impression. Hold the alginate impression over a vibrator on low or medium speed while the plaster is added, starting at the back of one side of the arch. The plaster should stream down the back of the impression. Add more plaster until it flows toward the front teeth to the other arch and out the other end, thus permeating the anatomical part of the model. Take the impression off the vibrator and pack the rest of the impression with plaster. Briefly vibrate the impression again for amalgamation. This is the anatomic portion of the model. If an art portion is to be added, the surface should retain small drops of plaster.

The dental assistant is responsible for preparing the art portion of the study model. Pour the anatomical portion of the study model and set it for 5 to 10 minutes. Clean the flexible rubber or disposable bowl to prepare it for mixing more plaster. The ratio of water to powder for the art portion is 40 mL per 100 grams of powder (thicker than the 50 mL/100gm used for the anatomical portion). Use a spatula to put the mixture on a glass slab or paper towel, creating a base. Turn the anatomical part of the model over onto the base and position it so that the tray handle is parallel to the slab or paper. Scoop surplus plaster along the edges to fill gaps. This is the two-pour method. The art portion can also be poured right after the anatomical part is filled by a single-pour technique. The model is allowed to set for 40 to 60 minutes, plaster on the outside of the tray is cut off with a laboratory knife, and the model is separated from the impression by holding the tray and lifting upwards.

Trimming Diagnostic Casts and Models

Don safety glasses. Wet the dry models in flexible mixing bowls. Ensure the base is parallel to the counter and occlusal plane. If not, trim it with the model trimmer. Apply even pressure on the trimming wheel, while supporting the hands on the trimmer table. Set the maxillary and mandibular models together in occlusion to examine further for parallelism. Once the two are parallel, draw a pencil line behind the retromolar area on the model. Trim the back of the model off perpendicular to the base. Reposition the two models in occlusion. Hold the two halves in place and cut off the untrimmed model at a right angle to its base, at the same spot as the opposing model. Draw lines as guides for trimming off the side areas, anterior cuts, and the heel portion. Trim the tongue area with a laboratory knife. Plaster fills the holes. Smooth with wet sandpaper. Apply model gloss. Polish the model and label it.

For side trimming, mark lines and make cuts on both models about 5 mm from and parallel to a line between the edge of the model and center of the premolars for the mandible, or the cuspids for the maxilla. Make anterior cuts on the maxillary model along a line from the midline to the area between the canine and cuspid on each quadrant. You may need to protrude the line outward, if teeth are in the way. For the mandibular model, make the anterior cuts back to each cuspid area in a more curved fashion. Heel cuts are small trimmed edges in the back on either side of each model that extend toward the center of the back.

Diagnostic casts are shown to the patient to explain treatment. They should be trimmed to specifications and look professionally prepared. Approximately two-thirds of the model should be the anatomical portion (1 inch) and the other third the art portion or base (½ inch), for a total depth of 1½ inches. Displayed in occlusion, the total height should be 3 inches. Each model should be symmetrically cut, using the angles described elsewhere. Casts placed in occlusion should be capable of maintaining that relationship when placed on their ends together. If they fall apart, they are not trimmed properly.

Articulator

Articulators are frames symbolizing the jaws. They are attached to study models to keep the models in occlusion and to move them. They are useful for examination of malocclusion. One of the most common types is the Stephan articulator, which is designed to demonstrate both up-and-down and sideways movements. It has hinges corresponding to the temporomandibular joints. A wax bite is placed temporarily to determine correct occlusion. The base of each model is scored, and then they are connected to bows on the device with additional impression plaster.

Dental Waxes

There are five categories of dental waxes: Pattern wax is composed of two hard waxes, inlay and baseplate. Inlay wax comes in dark sticks that are melted and placed on a die to create a pattern for a restoration, or heated to vaporization with the lost wax technique. Baseplate wax comes in sheets that are heated for use as denture bases.

Temporary processing waxes include soft boxing wax, sticky wax, and utility wax. Soft boxing was encloses impressions to keep gypsum in place. Sticky wax adheres to many types of surfaces when melted for temporary repair jobs. Utility wax has adhesive and malleable properties at room temperature, making it ideal for relieving patient discomfort. For example place it over orthodontic brackets to making wearing more comfortable.

Impression or bite registration waxes incorporate copper or aluminum particles. Hard blocks of study wax that can be whittled.

Undercut wax, which is placed in undercuts before making impressions.

Custom Trays

Custom trays are made from acrylic, resin, or a thermoplastic substance:

Self-curing acrylic tray resin - This system combines a polymer powder with a liquid catalyst or monomer, initiating polymerization and exothermic release of heat. Complete setting to a very hard state takes about a day.

Light-cured acrylic tray resin - Similar to self-curing acrylic, but remains malleable until a special curing light is activated, which initiates the polymerization and sets much faster.

(3) Vacuum-formed custom trays - These use heavy, stiff sheets of plastic resin. The resin is hung within a special unit and heated until soft. The sheet is then released onto the model, as vacuum pressure is applied.

Thermoplastic materials - Beads or buttons are softened and made pliant through exposure to heat, usually warm water. After shaping, hardening occurs as heat disperses.

A custom tray is fabricated to make an accurate impression. Therefore, the tray must be durable enough to hold the material during positioning and removal. It should be smoothed and shaped to the patient's arch. Ideally, it should allow the impression material to fill with consistent thickness in all regions of the arch. The tray should be adaptable to any type of dentition, from an edentulous condition to full dentition, and any other type of unusual area. Trays that have stops in the spacer to grip the impression material are a good design and provide greater accuracy for the impression.

The dental assistant adapts a working plaster or stone cast. The assistant draws a blue line in the deepest area of the entire margin. The assistant draws a red line for wax spacer placement 1 to 2 mm above the blue line. The red mark corresponds to about 2 to 3 mm below the tooth margin or above the lowest point of the vestibule, if edentulous. Spacers are made of pink baseplate wax, a special molding material, or wet paper towels. The assistant plugs any recessed undercuts in the model. The spacer material is heated, shaped, and trimmed to the red line with a laboratory knife. Stops or holes are cut at intervals on the top edges of the spacer to permit impression material through. The assistant drapes the top of the spacer with aluminum foil, if self-cured resin is being used to dissipate heat and facilitate removal of wax at the end of the procedure. Sometimes, the assistant paints a separating material over the spacer.

Self-Cured Acrylic Resin Custom Tray

The dental assistant mixes the self-curing resin components, the powder polymer and the liquid catalyst, in a wax-lined paper cup with a wooden tongue blade, until the mixture is uniform. Follow the directions from the manufacturer. The initial set or polymerization takes about 2 to 3 minutes. Apply petroleum jelly to your palms and the cast. The dental assistant takes the malleable resin and manipulates it into a doughy patty or roll for a maxillary or mandibular arch. A little is reserved to make a handle later. The resin patty or roll is inserted over and extending slightly beyond (1 to 2 mm) the wax spacer. For the maxillary tray, this means inclusion of the palatal area. The assistant manually contours it with a rolled edge. Use of the laboratory knife is permitted, but less desirable. The handle material is molded and attached to the front of the tray, near the midline, using a drop of the monomer catalyst liquid.

Don safety glasses. Remove the custom tray from the model and wax spacer after 8 to 10 minutes of setting. Remove the wax by melting or using a spatula, hot water, and a toothbrush. Trim the outside edges of the tray later, using an acrylic burr. Ensure the material is completely set (about 30 minutes). Clean disinfect, and label the tray. Before taking the impression, paint two thin coats of impression adhesive onto the inside of the tray and along the margins. Further secure the impression material by making holes in the tray with a round burr.

Vacuum-Formed Acrylic Resin Custom Tray

The dental assistant prepares the previously-made cast by immersing it in warm water for up to 30 minutes to remove surface air bubbles. Add spacers, if specified. Outline the outer margin. Place the cast on a vacuum-forming unit with a platform. Secure the unit between two frames with acrylic resin sheets. These hang above the platform. One of the frames contains a heating element. Turn it on to cause the resin sheet to droop downward. When the resin hangs down about an inch, the operator pulls the frames down over the cast, using the handles on the sides. Activate the vacuum right after the resin drops over the cast. Turn the heat off. Keep the vacuum on for a minute or two. Once the tray cools, take it off the frame. Release it from the model, and trim it to the preferred form with a laboratory scissors. Cut a handle and attach it using a torch. Clean, disinfect and label the tray.

Prosthodontics

Prosthodontics are artificial parts (prostheses) created in the dental laboratory to replace missing teeth or tissues. They can be fixed or removable. Fixed prostheses are designed to integrate into the natural dentition and are maintained through regular brushing and flossing. The purposes they serve include restoration of chewing ability, prevention of teeth movement by providing underlying support, speech improvement, promotion of oral hygiene, and for esthetic reasons. Crowns, inlays, outlays, bridges, and veneers are examples of fixed prosthodontics. The two categories of removable prosthodontics are partial dentures replacing one or more teeth in an arch, and complete or full dentures that take the place of all teeth in one arch. Partial dentures are held in place by underlying tissues and other teeth, while full dentures are supported by gingival and oral mucosal tissues, alveolar ridges and the hard palate.

Fixed prostheses are maintained by brushing and flossing. Toothbrushes selected should be soft, multi-tufted, and small enough to access all areas. Bridges can be cleaned by using a bridge threader to insert dental floss underneath. Interproximal brushes and tips are also available. Dental implants, which are titanium devices or screws that fuse with bone tissue by bonding (osseointegration), should be brushed with a similar type of brush and a specialized type of floss that is wider and designed to be wrapped around the implant (such as Proxi-Floss). Other maintenance measures include use of a plastic interproximal brush, water irrigators for plaque and debris removal, antimicrobial rinses, and a variety of plastic cleaning instruments. Removable prostheses or dentures are brushed with a special denture toothbrush and mild soap or toothpaste. Tissue under the denture should also be brushed. Dentures are removed and placed in cleaning agents to get rid of stains. Orthodontic devices should be maintained with specially designed toothbrushes, water irrigation, and an interproximal brush.

Patient Education & Oral Health Management

Preventive Dentistry

Good preventive dentistry is multifaceted. It involves daily brushing and flossing for removal of plaque and bacteria. Teach your patient correct techniques for brushing and flossing at the initial visit. It is advisable to use a disclosing agent at regular intervals to see how successful the removal has been. Children who are still developing dentition should undergo a fluoride program, including treatments at the office and in the home. A healthy patient should see the dentist every six months. Routine visits should include an examination, cleaning, and dental procedures, if indicated. In addition, good nutrition and adequate exercise have a positive impact on general health, including teeth and bones.

The oral health of infants is the responsibility of the parent or guardian. The adult removes the infant's plaque with an infant toothbrush or cloth while the child reclines. Instruct parents to bring the child to the dentist at age 3 years old. Preschoolers respond to visual instruction but they also have a short attention span. Role-play to teach the child oral hygiene habits. Tell the parent to oversee or perform tooth brushing at bedtime. Children ages 5 to 8 have a longer attention span and are eager for knowledge. They can be taught good oral hygiene techniques with visual aids, like short videos or pictures. Children ages 9 to 12, have an even longer attention span, greater curiosity, and the ability to brush and floss effectively on their own. They also have unique issues, such as peer group acceptance and dealing with mixed dentition, which the dental assistant should keep in mind when providing instruction.

Peer pressure and concern about personal appearance motivate all teenagers. Thirteen to fifteen-year-olds have poor coordination (due to growth spurts) and bad eating habits. Thus, they often have trouble with flossing. The decay rate in this age group increases dramatically. The dental assistant should give individualized instructions and encouragement to motivate young teenagers. Sixteen to nineteen-year-olds question authority and have busy schedules. The assistant needs to act more as a friend. Explain the processes involved in plaque and caries formation. Approach young and middle-aged adults on an individualized basis. Elder older than 60 have age-related concerns, such as tooth retention, disease-specific difficulties, maintaining oral hygiene with poor sight, or use of drugs that interfere with oral health. The professional needs to give advice based on each specific case.

Oral Hygiene Aids

Oral hygiene aids include disclosing agents, dentifrice, toothbrushes, flosses, mouth rinses, chewing gum, and a variety of interdental aids. Dentifrice is another term for toothpaste, used by the patient with a toothbrush or floss. Dentifrice products earn the ADA Seal of Acceptance if they are deemed both safe and effective. Toothpastes contain abrasive materials, and often fluoride for decay prevention, or other ingredients (for example whiteners or calculus inhibitors). Mouth rinses are designed to be swirled in the mouth to dislodge debris or temporarily get rid of halitosis, as adjuncts to brushing and flossing. Some have ingredients (alcohol) that eradicate microorganisms. Special oral hygiene gums chewed after eating carbohydrates encourage saliva production and loosen debris. Interdental aids clean between the teeth and stimulate the gums. They include the interproximal brush, dental stimulators, floss holders and threaders, and irrigators.

Interdental Aids

Interproximal brushes consist of a handle (often bent) attached to a small, nylon-bristled brush. They reach into interproximal areas, open bifurcations and trifurcations, and under orthodontic brackets. Dental stimulators activate soft tissues in interproximal areas and get rid of plaque. Some toothbrushes have rubber tipped stimulator ends. Wooden dental stimulators made of balsam wedges have plastic handles with toothpick tips attached; moisten both before use. Floss holders are "Y" shaped to hold floss for easy access to interproximal areas. Shift the floss up and down on the sides of the tooth and into the sulcus. Floss threaders are rigid plastic, shaped into a large loop at one end, through which floss is threaded. Insert the straight end into one side of the space. Pull it out the other for removal, leaving the floss for elimination of plaque and debris. A water irrigation device uses pulses of water to remove debris. Irrigators are for cleaning orthodontic brackets and prostheses and are ineffective against plaque.

Toothbrushes

All toothbrushes fall into two main categories: Manual or mechanical.. Manual toothbrushes have a head containing the bristles, an indented shank adjacent to the head, and a long handle. There may also be a rubber dental stimulator on the end. The head has a toe end at the exterior and a heel end at the interior. Bristle configurations differ on various brushes; they are usually spaced or multi-tufted. Manual toothbrushes with soft, nylon bristles are best because they are durable and will not wear away the teeth or gums. Mechanical toothbrushes are attached to a recharging unit or are battery operated. Their heads t can move in various directions: Reciprocating (back and forth), vibratory (quick back and forth), orbital (circular), arched (in a semi-circle), elliptical (oval rotation), or a combination of movements. Mechanical toothbrushes may also include sonic action.

Brushing Techniques

The main objective of tooth brushing is the thorough cleaning of every surface of all teeth. Manual brushing should take 2 to 3 minutes. Manual brushing techniques include the Bass, modified Bass, Charter, modified Stillman, rolling stroke, and modified scrub brushing techniques. Dentists most often recommend the Bass or modified Bass techniques because they are effective at removing plaque near the gums.

Bass technique: Hold the toothbrush bristles slanted at 45 degrees to the teeth, toward the gingival sulcus. Sequentially brush small areas, each for a count of 10, with small back and forth movements. Apply the toe bristles to the lingual surfaces of the front teeth. Modified Bass technique: Essentially the same, except after each area has been cleaned, bring the bristles are up over the crown toward the biting surface.

Charters and modified scrub brushing techniques are effective for plaque removal and gum stimulation. With the Charters brushing technique, the toothbrush head is pointed toward the end of the root. The brushes touch the gingiva, centered between adjacent teeth, and are aimed toward the teeth. Small areas are sequentially brushed for a count of 10 each, with small back and forth movements. Front teeth are brushed with the sides of the toe bristles and the brush parallel to the teeth. The modified scrub brushing technique uses back-and-forth movements centered initially between the gum and tooth. The brush is held perpendicular to the tooth surface. This is repeated until all teeth have been cleaned.

Modified Stillman and rolling stroke brushing techniques are effective for plaque removal and gingival stimulation. In both, the initial position of the bristles is toward the apex of the tooth. The modified Stillman method also positions the handle level with the biting surface. The bristles are brushed downward simultaneously, with a back-and-forth action, to cover the complete surface of the tooth for a count of 10. The patient performs a minimum of 5 sequences before continuing to the next tooth and repeating the sequence. With the rolling stroke brushing technique, the toothbrush is held parallel to the tooth, with the bristles toward the apex. The bristles are rolled from the gums down toward the teeth, including the biting surface. Each tooth is brushed in this manner 5 times before moving to the next one. A similar motion is applied on the lingual surfaces of the front teeth, using either the toe or heel portion.

Dental Floss

Dental flossing removes plaque and fragments from proximal tooth surfaces. Traditional dental floss comes as a thread that is either waxed or unwaxed. Waxed floss glides more easily and is less likely to tear or snag. Flosses can be flat tape, finely textured, colored, or flavored. Flossing requires 18 inches of floss. Secure the ends around the middle and ring fingers of each hand. Grasp a short section (about an inch) between the thumb and index finger of each hand. Draw the floss into each proximal space, using a gentle back-and-forth motion. In the maxilla, use both thumbs or a thumb and finger. For the mandible, use the two index fingers. The floss should be wrapped around the proximal surface and into the sulcus. Move the floss up and down along the surface for plaque removal. Transfer it to the proximal surface of the adjoining tooth, and repeat the action. Use a new section of floss for each space. Include the distal surface of the last molar.

Special Need Patients

All patients with special needs require empathy and individual attention from the dental professional. The nausea that usually accompanies pregnancy presents problems related to oral hygiene. Acid regurgitated from the stomach during bouts of nausea promotes decay, the act of tooth brushing often causes gagging, and the women commonly have bleeding gums. Advise your pregnant patients that these circumstances may occur, and suggest they perform dental hygiene when they are not nauseated. Cancer patients commonly experience xerostomia (mouth dryness), widespread caries (including the roots), gum bleeding, and deficient muscle function. Approaches to oral hygiene issues include use of topical fluoride and/or extra-soft or foam toothbrushes. Patients with heart disease experience similar problems. Patients with arthritis may need to use special large toothbrushes or floss holders.

Cariogenic Foods

Carbohydrates contain the chemical elements carbon, hydrogen and oxygen, and are comprised of sugars, starches and fibers. Carbohydrates from natural sources include fruits, grains, and legumes. Most naturally-occurring carbohydrates are not broken down to simple sugars until they arrive at the stomach. Cariogenic foods are converted to simple sugars right in the mouth, where bacteria changes them into acids. The acid demineralizes the enamel, predisposing the teeth to caries (decay). Manufactured sweets, such as candies and soft drinks, and naturally-occurring raisins and sticky fruits do are cariogenic. The dental assistant should evaluate the patient's diet for use of cariogenic foods. Explain the possible consequences to your patient. The acid from cariogenic foods can be somewhat neutralized if they are eaten with foods that stimulate saliva production. Conversely, eating cariogens late at night, when saliva production is low, enhances potential decay. New teeth in infants are susceptible to nursing bottle syndrome, rampant decay due to liquid sweets, such as fruit juice.

Diet

All food consumed by an individual is his diet. Nutrients are dietary chemicals, essential for growth, maintenance and healing. There are six classes of nutrients. Three are energy sources: Carbohydrates, fats, and proteins. The other three classes are vitamins, minerals and water. Carbohydrates (sugars, starches, and fibers) provide energy, so at least half of the diet should be carbs. Fats and lipids are water-insoluble and contain fatty acids. Fat insulates, transports Vitamins A, D, E and K, and provides energy when sugars are inaccessible. Proteins are linked amino acids. Proteins derive from plant and animal sources, and are vital for cell growth and repair. Of 20 possible amino acids, 10 are manufactured by the body and 10 are essential and must be provided in the diet. Animal proteins (eggs, milk, meat) contain all essential amino acids and are complete. Plant sources do not contain all essential amino acids and are incomplete. Different incomplete foods eaten in the same meal are complementary (e.g., beans and rice) and provide complete nutrition.

Consumed calories provide energy. Carbohydrates supply 4 Calories (C or Cal) per gram consumed, fats 9 Cal/gram, and proteins 4 Cal/gram. A person's rate of metabolism is the relationship between bodily changes and energy expenditure. Everyone has a resting or basal metabolic rate (BMR). BMR is higher in children, thin people, and expectant women. The primary energy source is carbohydrates, fats are also utilized when sugars are inaccessible. Conversely, if calories are not used, they are converted to fat and stored. Both carbohydrates and fatty acids comprising fats are made of the elements carbon, oxygen and hydrogen, in different configurations.

Vitamins

Nutrients that carry out essential functions but are not energy sources are vitamins. Four vitamins are fat-soluble and retained in the liver and other fatty tissues, Vitamins A, D, E and K. Vitamin A is available as carotene in dark leafy vegetables and orange or yellow fruits, and from dairy products and liver. It is essential for maintenance of mucous membranes, bones, skin (epithelial tissue),

and vision. Vitamin D or cholecalciferol is necessary for good bone and tooth growth. It is available in animal sources, such as eggs, liver, and fortified milk. It can also be produced in the body after ultraviolet ray or sun exposure. Vitamin E or alpha tocopherol is obtained via plant sources, such as avocadoes, wheat germ, almonds, and fortified margarine. It is an antioxidant that prevents other nutrients from breaking down. Vitamin K is found in green leafy vegetables and animal products, like milk, liver, and egg yolks. Its primary function is to stimulate the formation of prothrombin, which is involved in blood clotting and coagulation.

Vitamin C and B complex are water-soluble. Vitamin C (ascorbic acid) is found in all citrus fruits and vegetables, like tomatoes and broccoli. Vitamin C is a necessary component of collagen, needed in connective tissue. It prevents scurvy, aids wound healing, and helps tooth development. Vitamin B complex includes:
Thiamine (B_1), essential as a coenzyme in the oxidation of glucose and to avert the degenerative nerve disease beriberi

Riboflavin (B_2), which aids growth, energy release from food and protein production

Niacin (B_3) or nicotinic acid, needed for ATP synthesis and maintains the gastrointestinal and nervous systems Pyridoxine (B_6), which plays a role antibody, nonessential amino acids, and niacin production

Cyanocobalamin (B_{12}) synthesizes red blood cells (RBCs) and maintains myelin sheaths

Folacin is also essential for RBC production

Biotin and pantothenic acid help energy metabolism

All vitamins in proper amounts have beneficial effects. Vitamin A deficiency causes night blindness and inadequate bone growth.

Vitamin D deficiency causes rickets, osteomalacia, and inadequately developed teeth. Vitamin B_2 or B_6 deficiencies cause mouth fissures and inflammation of the tongue. Vitamin C deficiency causes scurvy with tooth loss and muscle cramps. Vitamin E deficiency causes RBC destruction. Vitamin B_{12} deficiency causes pernicious anemia.

Conversely, fat soluble vitamins, C, B_3 and B_6 are toxic if consumed to excess. Too much Vitamin A causes stunted growth and termination of menstruation. Vitamin C or D toxicity results in kidney stones. Vitamin E toxicity causes hypertension. Vitamin K toxicity causes hemolytic anemia or jaundice. Excess niacin causes rash and liver damage. Excess B_6 damages nerves. High amounts of other water-soluble vitamins are not toxic because they are excreted in the urine every four hours.

Minerals

Minerals are elements that cannot be broken down chemically. Seven major elements and a few trace elements are required to sustain life. Minerals with negatively or positively charged ions are electrolytes. Two major minerals, calcium and phosphorus, are important for development of bones and teeth and are necessary to prevent osteoporosis. Calcium is involved in muscle contraction, conduction of nerve impulses and blood clotting. Phosphorus is involved in energy transfer and pH balance. Milk and cheese are good sources of calcium and phosphorous. Sodium and potassium are complementary major minerals that maintain fluid balance in the blood. Sodium, found in table salt and processed foods, causes high blood pressure in excess. Table salt also contains the mineral chlorine, which helps pH balance. Sulfur is important because it is a necessary component of protein and plays a role in metabolism of energy. Magnesium, found mostly in green vegetables and whole grains, also affects energy metabolism.

Dietary Trace Minerals

Some minerals are found in the body in small or trace amounts.. Fluorine, which is necessary for strong teeth and to avert osteoporosis, is considered a trace element. Numerous trace minerals facilitate metabolic processes, including iodine, copper, chromium, selenium, manganese, and molybdenum. Iodine is unique in that is concentrated in the thyroid gland. The trace mineral iron is a carrier of oxygen in blood; a deficit of iron can cause anemia. Cobalt is also necessary for red blood cell maintenance. Zinc is required by the immune system and promotes tissue growth.

Prevention and Management of Emergencies

Emergency Kit

Each treatment room should have a self-contained oxygen inhalation unit (with a green oxygen tank) or a wall-piped system for nitrous oxide gas and oxygen. Test the oxygen tank(s) weekly. The dental office emergency kit should contain: Plastic or metal airways; tracheotomy needles; masks for cardiopulmonary resuscitation; tourniquets; sterile syringes; antihistamines to counteract allergic reactions; an Epi-pen (epinephrine); vasodilators like nitroglycerin to increase blood flow and treat high blood pressure (hypertension); a vasopressor, like Wyamine, to treat low blood pressure (hypotension); anti-convulsants, like Diazepam; atropine to block the vagal nerve and increase the pulse rate; and analgesics (pain relievers). Check the medications monthly for expiration dates. Replace when needed.

Oxygen Administration

The dental assistant can administer oxygen in emergency situations. A crash cart contains a green oxygen tank, masks, airways, a defibrillator, and resuscitation drugs. One crash cart should be available per floor; remember where it is located. Tell the receptionist to call an ambulance (911) and notify the dentist. Place the patient in the Trendelenburg position, lying on the back with feet raised above chest level. Position the oxygen mask over the patient's nose, with tubing to the side. Fasten the mask firmly. Administer oxygen without delay, at a rate of between 2 and 4 liters a minute. If the patient is still conscious, explain that he/she must breathe through the nose with the mouth closed. Try to calm and comfort the patient.

Cover the patient with a blanket to help prevent shock. The dentist or registered nurse intubates the unconscious patient and administers resuscitation drugs.

Adult Rescue Breathing

Rescue breathing in emergency situations may be performed by the dental assistant, hygienist, nurse, or dentist if the patient is orally unresponsive. Call Emergency Medical Services (911) before beginning. Gloves are suggested but not required. If the patient is not breathing, tilt the head back and raise the chin to open the airway. Look, listen and feel for breathing. If there is none, insert a resuscitation mouthpiece into the patient's mouth. Pinch the nose closed. Provide two breaths to make the patient's chest rise. If it does not rise, clear the blocked airway. Check the carotid pulse in the neck, using your middle and forefingers. Perform rescue breathing while there is still a pulse, one slow breath every five seconds for a minute, followed by a pulse check. Repeat the sequence until breathing is re-established or a more qualified person takes over. If the pulse stops, begin CPR. When the incident concludes, throw the mouthpiece into a biohazard container. Document the incident.

CPR

Cardiopulmonary resuscitation (CPR) is an emergency technique to revive a person whose heart has stopped beating. The process of CPR follows an ABC (and often D) pattern:
"A" represents the airway, which must be first be opened up to allow air flow
"B" signifies breathing, which the rescuer must observe and work to re-establish if the patient is not breathing
"C" stands for circulation, which the rescuer must check using the carotid pulse; if there is no pulse, then chest compressions interspersed with slow breaths are used to re-establish a pulse

"D" refers to defibrillation using an automated external defibrillator (AED) unit, if available

Dental assistants are legally required to recertify in CPR with the American Red Cross or the American Heart Association every two years at the Healthcare Provider Level.

Adult CPR

The dental assistant or dentist performs CPR on patients with cardiac arrest. The patient must be unresponsive, with no pulse or breathing. Call Emergency Medical Services (911) before beginning. Don gloves, if possible. Place the patient supine on the floor or flatten the dental chair. Look, listen, and feels for the patient's breathing. If there is none, open the patient's airway by inclining the head back and raising the chin. Place a resuscitation mouthpiece patient's mouth. Pinch the nose closed. Inflate the lungs with two breaths. Observe the chest's rise and fall. Check the carotid pulse for about 15 seconds. If no pulse is present, kneel beside the patient. Landmark the xiphoid process. Place your palms over the breastbone. Compress 15 times, followed by two breaths. After four cycles, check the carotid pulse again. Continue until the patient breathes or you are relieved by a rescuer with higher training. Discard the mouthpiece. Document CPR in the patient's chart.

Automated External Defibrillation

An automated external defibrillator (AED) can revive a person in cardiac arrest if it is applied within four minutes and damage is not extensive. Continue CPR until the unit is charged. You must be on a flat, dry surface. Connect the electrodes of the AED to the patient, as illustrated on the unit. Press the "analyze" button first for a readout, to ensure the unit is ready and electroshock is appropriate. Announce, "Stay clear of the patient." Restart CPR if defibrillation is contraindicated. The unit indicates by tone or light that it is ready to shock the patient. The AED display shows when defibrillation occurs. Test the pulse after the third shock. If there is a pulse, check the airway, breathing circulation and move the patient into recovery position. If there is no pulse, perform CPR for one minute before rechecking the pulse. If there is still no pulse, defibrillate again. Press the analysis button. Nine defibrillations can be performed. The unit indicates when to stop defibrillation.

Ambu Bag

An Ambu-bag is the proprietary name for a portable manual resuscitator or bag-valve-mask (BVM) device. Anytime a patient has an emergency involving respiratory failure or arrest, it is essential to deliver positive pressure oxygen to increase the relative amount of oxygen in the lungs, blood, and ultimately the brain. The preferred method is delivery of oxygen from a pressurized oxygen tank via a hose and mask. Emergencies occurring where an oxygen tank is unavailable can be addressed with an Ambu-bag, which has a self-inflating bag that fills up with air (and sometimes additional oxygen attached to a flexible mask), and seals to the patient's face. Positive pressure ventilation is delivered when the rescuer compresses the valve joining the bag and mask. Another portable method of resuscitation is a pocket mask, where the rescuer inflates the patient's lungs using exhaled air.

Intubation

Small dental tools and debris may dislodge in the patient's mouth during a procedure, causing obstruction. Intubation means placement of a tube into the airway to supply oxygen when the patient is unable to breathe independently due to obstruction. The dentist passes a long, curved Magill intubation forceps into the windpipe for endotracheal intubation and retrieval of objects obstructing the airway that are still visible. The assistant must be present to suction the mouth. Do not allow your patient to sit up during retrieval, as movement can result in further injury and force the object farther down the throat. If only one professional is present, or if the airway is partially obstructed, then tell the patient to bend his/her head down over the side of the chair and try to cough it free. Call 911. If full obstruction occurs, perform the Heimlich maneuver.

Foreign Body Airway Obstruction

A dental patient is reclined, anesthetized, and slippery objects are in the mouth, so there are many opportunities for foreign body airway obstruction (FBAO) to occur. The universal distress signal for FBAO is clutching of the throat with both hands. If the patient does this, suspend treatment immediately. A choking patient cannot speak. Breathing is difficult or absent. The mouth may be blue (cyanotic). Ask the patient to sit up and cough. If he/she cannot force out the foreign body independently, call for help. Perform the Heimlich maneuver to open the blocked airway. If the patient is conscious, stand behind him/her. Wrap your arms around the abdomen. Make one hand into a fist; grasp the other hand firmly over it. Deliver a series of swift subdiaphragmatic thrusts, until the airway is clear or the patient falls unconscious. The patient needs follow-up medical treatment in case the airway was damaged.

If a patient with foreign body airway obstruction (FBAO) becomes unconscious during the standing Heimlich maneuver, phone Emergency Medical Services (EMS) immediately. Brain death occurs in 4 to 6 minutes. Place the patient on his/her back. Don gloves. Lift the tongue and jaw and sweep the mouth with your fingers to remove the foreign body. Open the airway by tilting the head, lifting the chin, pinching the nose. Insert a resuscitation mask into the mouth. Blow two slow breaths into the airway. Repositioning of the head may be required. If the airway remains obstructed, then landmark the xiphoid process. Straddle the patient's thighs. Position the heels of both hands just below the xiphoid notch at the base of the sternum. One hand is on top of the other. Apply 5 abdominal thrusts, pressing toward the diaphragm. Continue thrusting until the airway is unblocked or EMS arrives to take over.

Syncope

Syncope is fainting, loss of consciousness from decreased blood flow to the brain and blood pooling in the extremities. Syncope is caused by stress, pain, shock from massive infection or drug reactions, or standing for too long. The patient faints because lying down restores bloodflow to the brain. The patient feels dizzy or nauseated, initially. Lower his/her head to increase bloodflow to the brain. If unconscious occurs but the patient is breathing normally, place him/her in the Trendelenburg position (lying back with slightly elevated feet), so blood streams back to the brain. If the patient does not breathe well, open the airway by inclining the head and raising the chin. Remove restrictive clothing (scarves or ties) or jewelry at the neck. Dispense oxygen, using an oxygen tank, mask, and tubing. If breathing does not resume in 15 seconds, remove the oxygen mask. Apply spirits of ammonia under the patient's nose with a gauze sponge for a second or two. The unpleasant fumes should stimulate the person to take in air and oxygen and revive within a minute. Call an ambulance and start CPR, if necessary.

Asthma

Asthma is a respiratory disease. It is often triggered by allergies or exposure to cold air, and is characterized by breathlessness and wheezing upon expiration. Asthma attacks are most likely to occur in the morning. A patient with asthma has narrowed bronchioles (small airways) in the lung. During exhalation, the lung collapses and bronchiole narrowing is exacerbated further, making it increasingly difficult to breathe. Administer antihistamines, such as albuterol, using an inhaler. The patient exhales first, and then inhales the bronchodilator drug through the device's mouthpiece, while depressing the canister portion. Bronchodilators expand the bronchioles to enhance airflow. Usually, two inhalations of bronchodilator will allay an attack and improve breathing in about 15 minutes. If not, dispense oxygen and call Emergency Services (911). Status asthmaticus is prolonged bronchial spasms, which can be fatal.

Allergic Reaction

An allergic reaction is a response to exposure to a foreign agent (antigen). The patient's immune system develops antibodies to the antigen. Subsequent exposures to the antigen set off an allergic or hypersensitivity response, in which large amounts of histamine and other chemicals are released. Mild allergic reactions include skin reddening (erythema) and hives (urticaria). Remove the irritant and dispense antihistamines. Chronic allergy produces eczema. Asthma is a moderate allergic response in the airways. Anaphylactic shock is a possibly fatal allergic reaction. Allergens in the bloodstream stimulate histamine release, causing an immediate depression in blood pressure, airway constriction, swelling of the throat and tongue, and stomach pain. Give epinephrine immediately with an Epi-pen in the thigh muscle. Call 911. Administer oxygen, if required. The patient needs hospital follow-up within 20 minutes.

Hyperventilation

Hyperventilation is deep and rapid breathing, usually as a result of anxiety. The patient who hyperventilates for a prolonged period becomes faint, looses feeling in the extremities, and cannot take complete breaths. Alkalosis (high blood pH) further exacerbates the anxiety and rapid breathing. Terminate the procedure. Sit the patient erect. Allay your patient's anxieties. Instruct your patient to hold his/her breath a few seconds before exhalation, which reverses the alkalosis by getting more carbon dioxide and less oxygen into the blood. Alternatively, have your patient breathe into a paper sack or their hands. The converse is shallow breathing or hypoventilation, which can result in CO_2 accumulation in the blood and needs supplementary oxygen by mask.

Epileptic Seizure

Epilepsy is a brain disorder, in which disorganized electrical impulses hop the hemispheres in a "storm". Epilepsy can occur through head injuries, drug withdrawal, high fever, and metabolic imbalances. Tonic/clonic seizures are convulsions. The obsolete term is grand mal. The patient jerks and twitches, becomes unconscious for up to 5 minutes, followed by incontinence and exhaustion. Prolonged convulsions are status epilepticus, which is potentially fatal. Call EMS. Absences are brief periods of blank staring and withdrawal. The obsolete term is petit mal. During partial seizures, an epileptic either retains consciousness (simple) or loses consciousness (complex). Both forms manifest as involuntary twitching; the main difference is recall ability. Petit mal and partial seizure do not require treatment. Stop the procedure. Remove all instruments from the mouth. After the seizure, place the patient on the right side with the airway open.

Type I and Type II Diabetes

Type I (juvenile) diabetes mellitus is a hereditary condition in which beta cells in the pancreas cannot produce insulin, a hormone that regulates glucose levels in the blood. Type I diabetics are insulin-dependent, meaning they must receive frequent injections of insulin to regulate blood sugar levels. Too much glucose in the blood is hyperglycemia, causing thirst, frequent urination, confusion, nausea, vomiting, abdominal pain, drunken behavior, and snoring. Too little glucose is hypoglycemia, with irritability, shaking, sweating, and loss of consciousness. Stop the procedure. Give the Type I diabetic his/her insulin pen or portable pump to prevent diabetic acidosis and possible coma. Type II diabetes mellitus patients have decreased sensitivity to insulin, with high blood glucose, obesity, and fatigue. Type II diabetes is probably not hereditary and tends to occur in adults. Type II diabetics can control their condition through diet and oral hypoglycemics. All diabetics have difficulty healing wounds.

Hypoglycemia

Hypoglycemia is too low a concentration of blood glucose (less than 70 mg/dl). It is caused by fasting, overexertion, stress, and drug reactions. Its symptoms are irritability nervousness, shaking, weakness, cold sweats, and hunger. Stop the procedure. Give 8 ounces of orange juice, or a glucose drink, or 6 glucose tablets, or 10 Lifesavers candies immediately. A delay may cause your patient to become unresponsive and require glucagon injections, or hospital treatment for acidosis. If the patient loses consciousness, call EMS (911) and apply a tablespoon of sugar to the buccal mucosa. Excess amounts of insulin can produce severe hypoglycemia and a critical drop in blood sugar, called insulin shock; in this case, intravenous glucose is indicated.

Angina Pectoris

Angina pectoris is chest pain. It indicates arterial damage and leads to heart attack if left untreated. Arteriosclerosis is hardening and narrowing of the arteries from plaque buildup, resulting in decreased bloodflow to the heart. Your patient may complain of chest pressure, or tightening, or a heavy weight behind the sternum. Pain may radiate up the neck or down the arms. If an episode of angina pectoris occurs in the dental office, stop the procedure. Check for increased blood pressure and pulse rate. Allow the patient to take sublingual nitroglycerin pills or spray to open up the coronary arteries and supply the heart with more oxygenated blood. Give the patient oxygen by mask. The patient can take up to three doses of nitroglycerin, spaced 3 to 5 minute apart, before you should consider it a myocardial infarction (heart attack) and must call 911.

Myocardial Infarction

A myocardial infarction (MI) or heart attack is an event in which a portion of heart tissue dies rapidly (necrosis), due to severe blockage or narrowing of the coronary arteries. The symptoms of MI are angina pectoris, ashen skin color, blue lips and ear lobes, and copious sweating. Chest pain from myocardial infarction cannot be assuaged with nitroglycerin administration, as with angina pectoris can be. If an MI occurs in the dental office, terminate the procedure. Call 911. Reposition the patient with his/her head slightly raised. Administer oxygen and nitroglycerine. Alleviate the patient's stress. MI is more prevalent in males, smokers, people older than 40, and diabetics. Heart disease can be controlled somewhat through diet, exercise, and lowering stress and blood pressure.

Congestive Heart Failure

Congestive heart failure (CHF) is eventually terminal. The heart is unable to pump sufficient blood to meet the needs of all organs. CHF affects five million people in the USA. Older adults are most at risk. Causes of CHF include previous heart attack, hypertension, coronary artery disease, cardiomyopathy, congenital heart defects, valvular disease, cardiotoxic drugs, myocarditis and endocarditis. Signs and symptoms are shortness of breath (SOB) when at rest or with exertion, chronic fatigue, edema, lung crackles and distended jugular veins. CHF patients need frequent bathroom breaks because they use diuretic drugs to increase urinary output and decrease fluid buildup and swelling.

Stroke

A stroke (cerebrovascular accident or CVA) is a sudden stoppage of blood flow to the brain. Strokes occur because a blood clot causes blockage (known as a cerebral embolism), or a blood vessel in the brain bursts (known as a cerebral hemorrhage). Vessel tissues in the brain die and cause a cerebral infarction. Signs and symptoms of stroke include severe headache, speech loss, dizziness, weakness or paralysis on one side of the body (hemiplegia), and loss of consciousness. If a patient experiences a stroke in the dental office, terminate the procedure. Remove all instruments from the mouth. Raise the patient's head slightly. Call EMS. Give oxygen by mask. Check vital signs until EMS arrives. Cardiopulmonary resuscitation may also be necessary.

Abscesses and Avulsed Teeth

Abscesses are pus-filled, inflamed cavities from bacterial infection. Abscessed teeth are hot and painful due to pressure and edema. Untreated infection spreads into the surrounding tissues, producing a fistula (passageway) leading from the oral cavity, which alleviates some of the pressure. The danger is infection of the meninges around the brain. Treatment is root canal therapy, removal of necrotic pulp, opening the pulp chamber, antibiotic therapy.

If the patient is conscious, wrap an avulsed permanent tooth in wet gauze and insert it between the teeth and lip. If the patient is unconscious or incapable, put the loose tooth in milk. Take patient and tooth to the dental office at once. The dentist then reattaches the tooth in the socket, using adjacent teeth to shore it up. Primary avulsed teeth are not reattached because infection or ankylosis (fusion of bone and cementum) can result. Primary teeth displaced to the side or loosened are repositioned and secured with a temporary splint as soon as possible.

Fractured Teeth

Broken teeth are addressed according the amount and type of breakage, the degree of discomfort, and age. The dentist usually gives a child with a broken tooth pulp treatment and a temporary restoration, with a follow-up assessment several months later. Tooth fractures involving the enamel alone need their rough edges smoothed. If the fracture involves both enamel and dentin, then the exposed dentin is covered with glass ionomer, calcium hydroxide, and a bonding agent for composite restoration. If the break extends down into the pulp, then pulp capping or removal is indicated. If the crown is cracked with exposure of pulp, then a root canal supplemented by posts and casts in the crown for stabilization and protection are probably necessary.

Soft Tissue Injuries

Soft issue injuries to the oral-facial area can occur easily during dental procedures because the oral cavity is damp and slippery, the patient may shift, or equipment can be dislodged. Soft tissue injuries to the area can also be caused outside the office by any contact with a sharp or dull object, electrical burns, or sports injuries. A situation unique to children is traumatic intrusion, the forcing of freshly erupted teeth back into their sockets after a tumble. Traumatic intrusion is treated by either permitting the teeth to re-erupt, or by moving them and using a splint across adjacent teeth for support. If traumatic intrusion occurs to primary teeth, the extent of damage to emergent permanent teeth underneath cannot be fully ascertained until they erupt.

Alveolitis

Normally, a blood clot forms over the socket where a tooth has been extracted. The clot protects the nerve endings and discourages infection. Alveolitis is a dry socket, where there is no blood clot formation, or the clot is rinsed out of the socket. Nerve endings are exposed and the extraction area is susceptible to infection. The therapy for alveolitis is cleansing with saline and stuffing the socket with a gauze strip or sponge drenched in the antiseptic iodoform to relieve pain. Analgesics may be used for palliation, such as ibuprofen. Medicated dressings are usually replaced in a day or two. In a surgical setting after extraction, anesthesia may be administered prior to alveolitis treatment.

Crowns

In addition to anatomical and clinical definitions of crown, the term also refers to prostheses that cover the coronal surface of a tooth with broad decay or other problems. There are full-cast crowns that enclose the complete coronal surface and partial crowns that cover up to three tooth surfaces. They are usually made of porcelain, gold, stainless steel, or a combination of porcelain and metal. Loss of a permanent or temporary crown is a dental emergency. A temporary fix is to use petroleum jelly or orthodontic wax to keep the crown in position. The individual must be careful during meals not to dislodge the crown. As soon as possible, the crown should be recemented in place with the appropriate type of cement.

Emergency Preparedness

The role of each person in the dental office during an emergency should be clearly identified in the job description and rehearsed. For example:
The front desk receptionist phones EMS, notifies the dentist, directs traffic, and reschedules patients
The assistant obtains the crash cart, provides first aid, and assists the dentist with life support
The hygienist provides first aid, and contacts the patient's next-of-kin and physician
The dentist leads two-person CPR and administers resuscitation drugs
Staff must cross train in various roles during routine practice drills, in case of absences or multiple casualties. Clearly post these emergency telephone numbers at Reception and in each treatment room: Emergency medical services (EMS); fire department; police; nearest hospital Emergency Room; oral surgeon; nearby doctor; Public Health; morgue. The universal emergency number is 911, except in some rural areas.

Topical Anesthetic Complications

Topical anesthetics can cause allergic and toxic reactions. Swelling, erythema, ulcerations, and difficulty swallowing or breathing up to a day or more after application indicate an allergic reaction, which should be treated with antihistamines. Toxic reactions are central nervous system (CNS) complications due to an overdose of topical anesthetic. The patient initially becomes talkative and anxious. His/her blood pressure and pulse rates increase, but later the patient becomes hypotensive and the pulse is weak and thready. Excessive administration of local anesthetic drugs can produce similar toxic reactions and paresthesia (numbness). Document reports of paresthesia because nerve damage can be permanent.

Drugs

Drugs are chemical that alter bodily processes, treat diseases, or alleviate pain. They are naturally-occurring or artificially created. Laws require certain drugs to be dispensed only by prescription, while others can be obtained over-the-counter (OTC). The only professionals licensed to write prescriptions for controlled substances are doctors, dentists, and physician assistants. The benefits of drugs must be balanced against their side-effects and drug interactions. Side-effects are inadvertent consequences of use of a particular drug. For example, the immunosuppressant drug cyclosporine, which thwarts organ graft rejection, makes the patient susceptible to infection. Drug interactions are unintentional consequences of simultaneous use of two or more drugs. The combination of drugs acts synergistically to magnify, diminish or change the effects of each. Drug addiction means physical dependency on a drug and withdrawal symptoms if it is discontinued.

Drug Laws

The Food and Drug Administration (FDA) controls drugs. Drug laws relevant to dental practice are the 1906 Pure Food and Drug Act, the 1938 The Pure Food, Drug, and Cosmetic Act, and especially the Comprehensive Drug Abuse Prevention and Control Act of 1970, which divides drugs into five schedules, based on their potential for abuse:
Schedule I drugs - great potential for abuse and no established medical benefit, such as heroin
Schedule II drugs - great possibility of abuse and dependence but with some known medical benefit, e.g., narcotics, opiates, some barbiturates, and amphetamines
Schedule III drugs - less potential for abuse and established medical utility; includes other barbiturates, stimulants, strong depressants, and combinations, including many drugs used in dental practice

Schedule IV drugs - some potential for abuse, with established medical utility, and little possibility of addiction; includes sedatives, anti-anxiety drugs, and certain depressants
Schedule V drugs - slight potential for abuse; dispensed over-the-counter

Drug Administration

These are the routes of drug administration in the dental office:
Oral as pills or liquids for prophylactic antibiotics
Topical administration for anesthesia (ointment or cream applied to the skin or oral mucosa)
Gas inhalation, particularly nitrous oxide
Injections: Intravenous (into the vein for rapid response); intramuscular (into muscle); subcutaneous (underneath the skin) or intradermal (between skin layers)
Sublingual (under the tongue, as with nitroglycerine and fentanyl)
Transdermal skin patch, releasing medication at a steady rate, as with nitroglycerine cream or nicotine patch
Rectal administration of suppositories or enemas may be applicable for patients at home before or after the procedure, e.g., Gravol for nausea or fentanyl for severe pain in cancer patients

Addictive Drugs

Tobacco, caffeine, and alcohol are readily available and legal for adults. However, all these drugs are addictive. Smokers and tobacco chewers are stimulated by nicotine, which predisposes users to lung, bladder and oral cancer, heart disease, stained teeth, gum damage, and halitosis. Moderate consumption of caffeinated drinks (coffee, tea, chocolate, maté, guarana) is safe, but excessive consumption overstimulates the heart and nervous system, creates stomach ulcers, and stains teeth. Alcoholic beverages contain ethyl alcohol, a depressant, which slows reflexes and leads to poor judgment, coordination, and speech. Chronic alcohol abuse lead to dependency, convulsions, delusional behavior, and cirrhosis of the liver.

Illegal Drugs

Two widespread illegal drugs are marijuana and cocaine.

Patients who have taken marijuana recently may have an extremely high heart rate. The active ingredient is tetrahydrocannabinol (THC), but marijuana is often dusted with contaminants, so it is equally a stimulant and depressant. Habitual use damages lungs and reproductive organs. Chronic marijuana users have problems with memory, speech, coordination, and lack of motivation. Currently there is no evidence of physical dependence on marijuana, but users become emotionally dependent on it. Marijuana reduces nausea in cancer patients and reduces eye pressure in glaucoma patients.

Cocaine is addictive both physically and psychologically. It is often combined with other addictive drugs, potentiating its effects and the possibility of drug interactions. It is a stimulant and numbs the mouth. Cocaine abuse leads to cardiovascular issues, extreme anxiety, violent conduct, mental illnesses, and death.

Narcotic Drugs

All narcotic drugs are depressants that have the potential for physical and psychological addiction. Two narcotics, morphine and codeine, are often administered as analgesics (pain killers). Morphine is for severe pain and may be administered intravenously, intramuscularly, or orally. Occasional use causes constipation, nausea, and disorientation. Habitual use leads to addiction. Codeine is for mild to moderate pain, usually in formulations with Aspirin or acetaminophen. Its main side effects are tiredness and constipation. Heroin has no accepted medical use. It is taken intravenously, subcutaneously, or via inhalation. Heroin addicts develop tolerance to high doses. Warning signs of heroin use are depressed respiratory and heart rates, constipation, and loss of appetite. A heroin overdose is an emergency situation, characterized by vomiting, diarrhea, shock, and loss of consciousness. Call EMS to transfer the overdosed heroin addict immediately to a hospital, where he/she can be given a narcotic antagonist.

Hallucinogenic Drugs

Hallucinogenic drugs are drugs of abuse. They cause a user to imagine events, people, or things that are not really present. Subsequently, the user has modified brain activity, causing unpredictable or violent behavior. LSD (lysergic acid diethylamide) and its close relative psilocybin are both hallucinogens. LSD is derived from the fungus ergot and psilocybin comes from mushrooms. Phencyclidine (PCP) is another hallucinogen that has both stimulatory and depressive effects, like violent conduct, convulsions, nausea, suppressed respiration, and prolonged memory loss. Mescaline, derived from the peyote cactus, does not promote such extreme behavior, but it can cause permanent psychosis. If you suspect your patient is abusing a hallucinogen, suspend treatment. Notify the dentist.

Amphetamines and Barbiturates

Amphetamines and barbiturates have opposite effects, but both are addictive. Amphetamines are stimulants, increasing heart and respiratory rates and blood pressure. Aggressive behavior and poor judgment are warning signs of amphetamine use. Amphetamines do have an accepted medical use in treatment of narcolepsy or for attention deficit hyperactivity disorder (ADHD). Barbiturates slow down brain activity and have a calming or tranquilizing effect. Phenobarbital is administered for insomnia, epilepsy, and anxiety (including in the dental office). The main issues with barbiturates are dependency and tolerance with long-term use, withdrawal symptoms if taken away after prolonged use, and potentially critical overdosing. Overdosing causes disorientation, coma and death.

Antibiotics

Antibiotics treat bacterial infections. Broad-spectrum antibiotics kill many microorganisms, including helpful normal flora. Penicillin, and its derivatives amoxicillin and ampicillin, are broad-spectrum antibiotics. An antibiotic can only kill organisms sensitive to it; many organisms are now resistant due to overuse of antibiotics. Antibiotics can cause allergic skin or respiratory reactions, which are treated with antihistamines. Common antibiotic side-effects are nausea, diarrhea, and yeast infections due to disruption of normal flora. Prophylactic ampicillin taken 2 hours before teeth scaling prevent heart complications (for bacterial endocarditis) in patients who had rheumatic fever. The penicillin derivative oxacillin is for Staphylococcus aureus infections. Penicillin G is only for Gram-positive bacteria. People with penicillin allergies are generally given erythromycin, instead. Tetracyclines are antibiotics that discolor emerging teeth and precipitate kidney failure.

Dental Drugs

Anticholinergic drugs block nerve impulses. They reduce lung secretions while the patient is under general anesthesia, treat bradycardia, and dilate the pupils of the eyes. Dentists give anticholinergics to inhibit the patient's salivation while an impression is made. The drugs of choice are atropine sulfate or propantheline bromide.

Any drug that relieves pain but does not cause unconsciousness is an analgesic. Non-narcotic analgesics include ibuprofen and acetaminophen; they are for mild to moderate pain. Narcotic analgesics produce stupor and sleep and are for moderate to severe pain. Dental narcotics include morphine sulphate and meperidine hydrochloride. Aspirin is avoided because it inhibits healing due to its blood-thinning and clot-suppressing qualities. It also irritates the stomach.

Tranquilizers, particularly diazepam (Valium), are often given prior to procedures to relax anxious patients.

Blood

Blood transports nutrients, antibodies, drugs, and diseases throughout the body. Blood helps to regulate body temperature and pH. Antibodies and white cells (leukocytes) in blood protect against infection. Clotting factors and calcium in blood protect against injury. Blood is 55% liquid plasma and 45% formed elements. The three types of blood corpuscles are:
Erythrocytes (red cells or RBCs) containing the oxygen carrier protein hemoglobin
Leukocytes (white cells or WBCs) that fight disease
Thrombocytes (platelets) involved with blood clotting
People with blood dyscrasias have misshapen corpuscles or imbalanced blood elements. Dental assistants must beware hemophilia, a hereditary lack of clotting Factor VIII that causes the male patient to bleed uncontrollably with the slightest injury. Leukemia, a progressive blood cancer in which abnormal leukocytes grow uncontrollably, causes the lymph nodes to swell. Hence, the dentist may be the first practitioner to diagnose leukemia.

The patient who experiences significant blood loss needs intravenous fluid and electrolyte replacement, and perhaps a blood transfusion. If the dentist books a procedure where hemorrhage is likely, then the Blood Transfusion laboratory crossmatches the patient beforehand. Two units of blood are reserved in the laboratory's refrigerator, in anticipation of hemorrhage. For example, males with hemophilia or Christmas disease and females with von Willebrand disease may need immediate transfusions, additional clotting factors, and IV fluids. Book a registered nurse to assist with the procedure. The blood group (A, B, AB, or O) and Rh type (negative or positive antigen) of both donor and recipient must match before transfusion. A fatality can occur from mismatched blood causing hemolysis. Postpone the dental procedure if an exact match cannot be found. O– individuals are universal donors, in great demand. AB individuals are universal recipients (the rarest and most difficult group to match).

Viral Hepatitis

Hepatitis is inflammation of the liver, characterized by jaundice, abdominal pain, fever, and weakness. Hepatitis A and E are caused by contact with contaminated food or water, and usually just produce temporary flu-like symptoms. People with Hepatitis A are treated with gamma globulin injections or the Havrix vaccine. Hepatitis types B, C and D are bloodborne. Hepatitis B is quite virulent and some forms are fatal in 14 days. All dental personnel should be vaccinated against it with Heptavax-B, Recombivax HB, or Energix B in a sequence of three injections. Hepatitis C is less virulent but more chronic; vaccine development is impeded by its mutational ability. Both Hepatitis B and C may present asymptomatically, as jaundice, loss of appetite, abdominal discomfort, fever, muscle pain, or weakness. Hepatitis D can only replicate in conjunction with Hepatitis B. Dental personnel must wear PPE and avoid contact with body fluids of patients with hepatitis.

HIV

The human immunodeficiency virus (HIV) is transmitted via sexual intercourse, from mother to fetus, or through transfusion with infected blood products. The retrovirus replicates in the immune cells called T-lymphocytes, so they cannot alert the body to infection. Some HIV carriers are asymptomatic, while others have ambiguous conditions like weight loss, night sweats, or diarrhea. HIV infection precedes AIDS, acquired immunodeficiency syndrome, characterized by dementia and opportunistic infections like thrush, pneumonia, and Kaposi's sarcoma. AIDS is incurable but there are now several classes of drugs that slow its effects, including reverse transcriptase and protease inhibitors. Life expectancy has risen from 18 months to 10 years for many AIDS patients. The most commonly used drugs are zidovudine (AZT) and acyclovir. Dental personnel must wear PPE and avoid contact with body fluids of patients with HIV or AIDS.

Ulcers

Many oral ulcers or sores are not contagious and can be soothed with topical anesthetics. Cold sores are contagious, and are caused by herpes simplex virus type 1 or 2 (HSV1 and HSV2). Herpetic lesions are vesicles filled with fluid containing virus. Lip clusters of these sores are termed herpes labialis. Herpes viruses attach to nerve cells and remain in the body for life. Herpes virus is usually dormant, but is reactivated by exposure to stressors or acidic food. The dental team should avoid contact with cold sores. Reschedule the patient if you notice lesions are present, if possible. If procedures must be performed during an active infection, topical treatments can provide some relief. Wear gloves and other PPE. If the patient's vesicles break, the dental worker can get crusty ulcerations on his/her hands called herpetic willow.

Bacterial Endocarditis

Bacterial endocarditis is inflammation of the lining of the heart caused by a bacterial infection. Patients with a history of congenital heart disease or rheumatic fever are very susceptible to bacterial endocarditis. People who have had heart valve replacements, joint replacements, or organ transplants are also predisposed to development of bacterial endocarditis. An individual with a heart murmur is at risk for endocarditis. Insertion of dental implants also puts patients at risk. Any patient with one of these risk factors should be given a broad spectrum antibiotic prior to dental treatments or procedures to avoid infection. The recommended standard prophylactic course of therapy for adults is pre-procedure oral amoxicillin V (3 gm 1 hour before), erythromycin stearate (1 gm 2 hours before) or Clindamycin (300 mg 1 hour prior) followed by half doses 6 hours later. Doses for children depend on body weight: 50 mg/kg amoxicillin, 20 mg/kg for erythromycin, or 10 mg/kg for Clindamycin given 1 hour before procedures, followed by half doses 6 hours later.

Office Management Procedures

Dental Practice Act

Every state has a Dental Practice Act, which outlines the legal constraints and controls, which the dental team members must follow. Each state has a board that administers the Dental Practice Act, usually the State Board of Dental Examiners or the Dental Quality Assurance Board. The state board issues a dentist, a hygienist, and usually a dental assistant, a license to practice in that state only if they meet certain minimum qualifications. These requirements include educational qualifications, moral requirements, and successful completion of a written examination. A license to practice can be used in another state if the two states have a reciprocity agreement. The board defines reasons for suspension or revocation of a license. The Dental Practice Act and the corresponding board define which expanded functions a dentist can delegate to a dental assistant. Most often, the Doctrine of Respondeat Superior is invoked, making the dentist ultimately responsible, but leaving the employee accountable, too.

General Certification Requirements

Not all states require national certification for dental or orthodontic assistants. The Dental Assisting National Board, Inc. (DANB) offers written or computerized examinations for national certification. The CDA or Certified Dental Assistant exam has three parts: General Chairside (GC), Radiation Health & Safety (RHS) and Infection Control (ICE). The COA or Certified Orthodontic Assistant exam has two parts: Orthodontic Assisting (OA) and the ICE, both of which must be passed within a five-year period. Yearly continuing education and renewal is required for maintenance. Many states require DANB or some other type of licensure for performance of certain functions. DANB also administers examinations for the Certified Dental Practice Management Administrator (CDPMA) exam.

Certified Dental Assistant Examination

There are three possible pathways a candidate can take to the CDA examination or the General Chairside (GC) component through DANB. All three pathways require the candidate to have earned DANB-accepted cardiopulmonary resuscitation (CPR) certification within the previous two years. The candidate can write the Radiation Health & Safety (RHS) and Infection Control (ICE) examinations without the following prerequisites:
Pathway I requires graduation from an ADA-accredited program for dental assisting or hygiene
Pathway II requires a high school diploma, or equivalency, with 3,500 hours of documented work experience as a dental assistant, either full-time over two years, or a combination of full and/or part-time within four years
Pathway III means the candidate is currently or was previously a DANB CDA or has a dental degree (DDS, DMD or foreign)

Jurisprudence, Contracts, and Torts

Jurisprudence is the legal system set up and enforced at various governmental levels. Laws that pertain to dentistry are referred to as dental jurisprudence. There are both civil and criminal laws. Civil laws are more often invoked in the dental setting, as they pertain to either contracts or torts. A contract is an enforceable covenant between two or more competent individuals. An agreement between a dentist and his or her patient is a contract. It can be an expressed contract, with written or verbal terms, or it can be an implied contract, where actions create the contract. Tort law governs the other branch of civil law. Torts relate to standards of care and wrongful actions that cause injury to a patient. Criminal laws speak to crimes that endangers society in general. There are occasions when criminal law may apply to

- 84 -

dentistry, usually resulting in fines, incarceration, and discipline by the state dentistry board.

Contract Law

There is an expressed or an implied contract between the dentist and patient. The dental assistant or other personnel are the dentist's agents. The dentist is ultimately responsible for breach of contract under the Doctrine of Respondeat Superior. Nevertheless, the assistant's words or actions regarding care are legally binding upon the dentist. Breach of contract is failure to fulfill and complete the terms of the contract. There are four situations where a contract can be legally abandoned:
The patient releases the dentist by failure to return for treatment; ideally, the patient sends the dentist a certified letter of discharge, but this is not required
The patient/guardian does not comply with specific instructions from the dentist regarding care
The patient no longer requires treatment
The dentist formally withdraws from the case by sending a certified letter to the patient explaining the situation, to preclude any charges of patient abandonment.

Standard of Care

Standard of care is covered by tort laws. Dental specialists are expected to provide due care, the accepted reasonable and judicious care. Malpractice is professional misconduct, resulting in failure to provide due care. Most malpractice lawsuits are related to professional negligence, the failure to perform what is considered standard care. Tort laws pertain to unethical or immoral behavior by the professional, resulting in harm to the patient. Examples are defamation of character, invasion of privacy, fraud, and assault and battery. Defamation of character harms an individual's character, name, or reputation through untrue and malicious statements, either written (libel) or spoken (slander). Invasion of privacy is

unsolicited or unauthorized exposure of patient information. Fraud is intentional dishonesty for unfair or illegal gain. Assault is declaring your intent to touch a patient inappropriately. Battery is the actual act of inappropriate touching. People who provide unpaid assistance to the injured in emergency situations are protected from assault and battery charges under the Good Samaritan Law.

Americans with Disabilities Act

In 1990, the federal Americans with Disabilities Act (ADA) was passed by Congress. It mandates that people with disabilities cannot be discriminated against in terms of employment and access to public services, accommodations, and goods. ADA provided more sophisticated telecommunication services to facilitate the hearing and speech impaired. ADA requires dental offices to have ramps, entryways, and treatment rooms that provide access and accommodate the needs of the disabled. Your office must have at least one accessible room where patients in wheelchairs can be positioned for dental procedures. Technically, ADA applies to facilities with more than 15 employees, but all dental offices should strive to comply with ADA.

Dental Records

A patient's dental record must be correct and current because it is a subpoenable court document that may be reviewed by a judge, prosecutor, defense lawyers, and privacy commissioner. You may be required to appear in court to explain your documentation. Document all care and payments legibly in ink. If you make a mistake, never use correction fluid or an eraser to fix it. Strike through the original entry with one line. Write the correct information above it. Initial and date the change. Keep records at least seven years from the last service date. Most dentists keep them indefinitely because of variations in the statute of limitations, the time period for local legal action. Place a signed informed consent in the chart for any surgical procedures. The dentist must explain the procedure, risks, expected results, alternatives, and perils associated with denying treatment before asking the patient to sign the informed consent form. Implied consent is an implicit contract between dentist and patient whenever the latter allows work to be performed.

Ethics

Ethics are moral principles or values indicative of the times. The American Dental Association's Principles of Ethics outlines the values that you must adopt to stay in practice. The main ethical concerns relate to advertising, professional fees and other charges, and the responsibilities and entitlements of the dentist relative to the patient. Dental advertising is presently considered ethical, providing it is truthful. Up until the 1980s, advertising was considered crass. Ethical behavior related to professional fees and charges means your firm's billing must conform to what other local dentists charge, the charges must be correct, and insurance dealings and missed appointments can be charged. Current ethics dictate that the dentist cannot refuse to see a patient based on discrimination against race, religion, or HIV status. HIV-infected dentists must limit their work to procedures and techniques that will not infect others. It is unethical for the dentist to be swayed by financial gains.

HIPAA

HIPAA is the federal Health Insurance Portability and Accountability Act of 1996. Congress ratified HIPAA to safeguard electronic healthcare communications, including claims, funds transfers, eligibility and claims status inquiries and replies. HIPAA directed the Department of Health and Human Services (HHS) to implement national standards for clerical and financial electronic transmissions related to healthcare. Dentists and all other healthcare providers and health plans must comply with HIPAA's privacy standards by protecting health information and the patient's rights. To find out the latest guidelines for dental offices, parameters related to use and disclosure, enforcement and preemption, visit http://www.hipaa.org/.

Protected health information (PHI) is any patient identifier, such as name, Social Security number, birth date, or address. Cover all records in the reception area, so they cannot be seen by patients and visitors. Lock up unattended records. Play quiet background music to blur phone conversations, and be discrete. Place computer screens and fax machines out of patient viewing areas. Disguise names with bar codes, so the individual cannot be identified, before open transmission. Each dental office appoints a privacy officer (PO) who is responsible for informing patients about their privacy rights. HIPAA grants patients the right to access and copy their own dental information. Each dental office must have a written PHI policy, including requirements for use and disclosure of patient information and procedures for handling grievances. Information released to third parties must be preauthorized by the patient and kept to a minimum. Violations of PHI under HIPAA are punishable by up to $250,000 in fines and 10 years imprisonment.

Your staff manual must include HIPAA's minimum requirements:
Table of contentsThe privacy officer (PO) in charge of informing patients about their privacy rights
Job descriptions of all personnel, to establish who has access to patient's information
Privacy policy statement
HIPAA training plan with training schedule
Copies of HIPAA forms regarding compliance, documentation, and the scheme for reporting violations
Confidentiality agreements between the dentist and patient
Agreements between your office and business associates, such as dental laboratories,

computer services, records shredder, temporary employment agencies, and trash removal company
Contingencies for change

ADAA

There are 17 pledges that members of the American Dental Assistants Association (ADAA) subscribe to in their Code of Professional Conduct. The pledges are primarily related to ethics. Many of these relate to the relationship between the dental assistant and the Association, such as the dental assistant will:
Abide by the bylaws and regulations
Maintain loyalty to the Association
Follow Association objectives
Respect members and employees, serve, and act cooperatively with them
Refrain from spreading malicious information regarding the ADAA
Utilize sound business principles related to the organization;
Serve the Association and instill public confidence in it
Uphold high personal standards of conduct
Hold separate personal opinions from those endorsed by the ADAA
Refrain from acceptance of compensation from other members
Try to influence relevant legislation in a legal and ethical way

Daily Routine

Every morning, the dental assistant changes from street wear into protective clothing, like a lab coat or uniform, so that external contaminants do not enter treatment rooms. The assistant then turns on the : Lights; dental units; vacuum system; air compressor; x-ray processors; sterilizers; communication system; and computers. The assistant checks the patient schedule and performs routine housekeeping chores, like: Unlocking files; organizing the reception and business areas; replenishing water and solutions for radiographic processing; preparing disinfectant solutions; setting out trays and

lab work for the first patients; and restocking any necessary supplies. The assistant finishes any overnight sterilization procedures before the dentist needs the instruments.

Ideally, two dental assistants participate in closing the office every day. They need to clean the chairs and units in the treatment rooms, flush various systems, and shut off switches. They process, mount, and file x-rays, and turn off radiographic processing equipment and the safe light. One assistant sterilizes used instruments while the other sets up trays for the next day. One assistant verifies that all laboratory work was sent out, and completed lab work has been returned. They deal with assigned chores, like insurance, bookkeeping, confirming appointments, and pulling charts for the next day's appointments. They turn off all business equipment, turn on the answering machine, and bolt windows and doors. Assistants change out of their uniforms into street wear before leaving, so they do not bring contaminants home.

Treatment Room Preparation

The dental assistant is responsible for preparing the treatment room between patients. This includes cleaning, disinfecting, and placing barriers on all areas (including charts) that may be touched. The Infection Control (ICE) exam covers appropriate procedures. The assistant pulls the rheostat, chairs, and mobile carts out of the patient's pathway, and lifts up the dental light. The dental chair should be about 15 to 18 inches above the floor, with the arm positioned for patient access. The dental assistant reviews the chart and sets out any needed radiographs, trays or lab work.

Patient Preparation

After preparing the treatment room, the assistant then greets the patient by name in the reception area and escorts him/her to the treatment room.. The assistant illustrates where to put personal items. The assistant offers mouthwash, tissues for lipstick removal, a lip lubricant, and a drink of water to the patient and then seats him/her in the dental chair. The dental assistant puts the bib apron on the patient and gives him/her safety glasses to wear. The assistant asks about changes in the medical history, and inquires whether the patient has any questions. The assistant places the most recent radiographs on the view box. The assistant positions the patient supine for treatment, with the headrest supporting the head. The assistant adjusts the rheostat, operator's chair, assistant's stool, and lamp. The assistant dons a mask and protective eyewear. After washing his/her hands, the assistant dons gloves, then sets up trays, saliva ejector, air-water syringe, evacuator, and handpieces.

Patient Dismissal

After the operator has finished the dental procedure, the dental assistant is responsible for rinsing and evacuating the patient's mouth. The assistant pulls the dental light aside, positions the dental chair to upright, removes fragments on the patient's face, and takes off the bib. The assistant instructs the patient to stay seated for a minute, in case he/she is dizzy as a reaction to anesthetic. The assistant places the used bib, evacuator, air-water syringe tips, and saliva ejector on the tray. The assistant either takes off the treatment gloves and washes his/her hands, or uses overgloves to immediately record procedures performed on the chart or electronically. The assistant collects the chart and radiographs. The assistant provides the patient with postoperative instructions and returns his/her personal items. The assistant leads the patient to the receptionist, who deals with later appointments and payments.

Dental Receptionist

The dental receptionist is responsible for initially greeting patients, helping them to fill out needed paperwork, answering the telephone, taking memos, arranging appointments, overseeing the charts and records, and other assigned tasks. The receptionist may or may not assume the role of dental office bookkeeper.

Patient Scheduling

Patient scheduling is performed by the receptionist. Appointment books are being phased out in favor of computer software. However, all personnel should know how to schedule and cancel an appointment with the correct color-code manually and on computer, in case the system fails or requires maintenance. Ten or 15-minute blocks are allocated for expected procedures. Include some time with the dental assistant alone and in tandem with the dentist. Allow double booking when one professional is free to attend to another patient's needs. Block out dates when the dentist is unavailable throughout the year on an appointment matrix. Set aside buffer times in the morning and afternoon for dental emergencies. Schedule children around their nap times or school hours. Make considerations for patients with special needs, such as booking an interpreter or attendant.

Appointment Book Entries

Determine an appropriate time in conjunction with the patient. Use a pencil for appointment book entries to allow for changes. Enter the patient's name, phone number, age (for children), type and length of appointment. Give the patient an appointment card immediately. Familiarize the receptionist with the length of various procedures, to avoid downtime, overtime, scheduling conflicts, and double booked treatment rooms. Schedule contagious patients at the end of the day. Sales representatives require appointments. Students must work when qualified staff are available to supervise them. If you rely solely on computer bookings, print off the next day's schedule in case of computer failure.

Telephone Etiquette

All personnel should be aware of good telephone etiquette:
Remember, patients and visitors in the waiting room can overhear your conversation, so be discreet
Answer all incoming calls within 2 to 3 ringsThe practice to the caller, e.g., "XYZ Dental Clinic. [Your name] speaking. How may I help you?"
Be organized, attentive and courteous. Speak clearly and directly into the mouthpiece, pronounce words properly, and speak at a normal speed.
Practice good listening skills
Obtain and use the caller's name
Screen the call; find out where to direct it best
Take a message, including date, time, caller's name, phone number, recipient's name, the communication, and callback parameters
Do not keep a caller holding longer than one minute
Reserve outgoing calls primarily for next day appointment confirmations
When communicating with patients whose primary language is not English, be patient, speak slowly at a normal volume, and repeat if required. Get an interpreter when necessary.

Communication Technologies

Voice mail changed the way dental offices operate, because the system automatically routes the caller to the mailbox for a specific professional, without screening by a receptionist. You are legally responsible for ensuring patients can access dental personnel in an emergency. Do not let an emergency caller flounder in "voice mail jail". List the numbers for the locum tenens and nearest emergency dental clinic in the outgoing message on your answering machine. Turn the machine on only when personnel are not present. Check for messages as soon as you return. An answering service operator can contact the dentist via a pager that flashes the patient's callback number. If the call is unanswered in a pre-agreed time, the service reroutes the call to the locum tenens. Healthcare professionals may carry cellular phones for direct contact, and some are capable of receiving faxes, images, and text messages. Answering services and cell phones are more expensive than voice mail, but help ensure legal compliance with duty of care.

Computers

Most dental business office systems are at least partially computerized. Networked personal computers (PCs) are connected to a secure server that complies with HIPAA. The computer programs most used are for word processing, x-ray imaging, spreadsheets, accounting, and database management. Microsoft Works, ABLEdent, Dentrix, and DentiMax are examples of common dental office software. Database management is particularly important in a dental office because these programs store vital patient contact and insurance information, track and analyze data. Your practice needs an Internet Service Provider (ISP), antivirus software, a firewall, and an e-mail account regularly monitored by the receptionist.

Dental office computers must comply with HIPAA regulations. Safeguard against computer viruses and hackers with regular antivirus and firewall updates. There must be an audit trail or another way to ensure only authorized personnel access patient records. Back up data daily to disc or external hard drive. Off-site storage is safest, in case of fire or flood. Computer operators must practice good ergonomics to avoid repetitive strain injuries, like carpal tunnel. Position the monitor with the top just below eye level and at a slightly backward incline. Position the keyboard at a height that allows for relaxed shoulders and flat wrists. Sit in a chair with lumbar supports, armrests low enough that they are not used during keyboarding, and a shallow seat to permit leaning backwards. Sit with your thighs at or just above your knees, feet firmly planted on the floor, and head directly over your shoulders. Protect yourself from eyestrain with an anti-glare screen and by looking away from the computer for 10 minutes every hour.

Patient Recall Methods

Patients are scheduled for continued care or recall appointments by one of four methods: Set the computer to automatically generate a recall date and inform the patient at the end of the visit.

At month end, the computer generates a list of patients for recall the next month, and the receptionist contacts them.

Schedule a tentative recall in the appointment book six months in advance while the patient is in the office, and tell him/her to confirm the appointment when the date nears.

Ask the patient to self-address a postcard. Place it in a chronological card file by month. Mail the card to the patient two weeks before ideal recall.

Color-code an index card with all pertinent patient information. Phone all patients with the same color code one month beforehand.

Dental Records

Keep dental records in color-coded file-folders. File cabinets must be locked when unattended to comply with privacy laws. The most popular type of file cabinet used in dental offices is the open-shelf lateral file cabinet, in which files can be pulled out. Vertical file cabinets are often used. Files must be sorted alphabetically, starting with the last name, proceeding to the first name, and lastly the middle name. Patient information sent via computer or facsimile must be protected from hackers. Keep records indefinitely. Microfilm records older than seven years. Keep a tickler file containing index cards with tasks that should be completed by a certain time. Alternatively, set a computer reminder to perform the tasks.

Patient Fees

Dental offices set up a fee schedule for specific services rendered. Fees charged are defined as usual, reasonable, or customary. The usual fee is that normally charged by the dentist. A reasonable fee is one falling in the midrange charged, based on the procedure and difficulty. The customary fee reflects local averages up to the 90th percentile. Insurance companies will not reimburse amounts above what they have determined to be usual, reasonable and customary. When a dentist charges less, for example, as a professional courtesy or for a limited insurance program, there is no source to recover the rest of the usual, reasonable or customary fee.

Bookkeeper

The employee hired to be the dental office bookkeeper deals with all office finances, including Accounts Receivable (money owed to the practice) and Accounts Payable (for which the office owes money). The bookkeeper may also handle dental insurance, payment arrangement details, and the inventory and supply system. Many dental offices have an office manager who coordinates and provides backup for these duties.

The dental office bookkeeper handles Accounts Receivable and Accounts Payable, either by computer software or the manual pegboard system. Computerized systems have all pertinent patient information, description of services, charges, payments, and insurance information organized and easily accessible. The account status can be viewed or printed out. The pegboard system uses day sheets that list patient names and all procedures, charges and receipts for that day. No-carbon-required paper is used. There are columns for balancing all daily and individual patients' Accounts Receivable. Total amounts received daily are deposited promptly in a bank account. Patients are invoiced monthly. Partial or deferred arrangements are extended to patients with good credit ratings.

Dental Insurance

A person who has contracted dental insurance is the subscriber. Anyone covered by the policy is a beneficiary. Insurance can be primary or secondary, depending on whether it is obtained via a subscriber or spouse. Group plans are offered by an employer to its employees, or by an organization to its members. Individual plans are available to members of the public. Dependents are spouses, children younger than 18 years old, or full-time college students. A carrier is the insurance company administering the plan. Carriers set annual maximums for reimbursement and deductible amounts that must be paid before benefits accrue. Predetermination of benefits is a process by which the dentist sends a proposed treatment plan to the carrier to calculate how much it will covered.

Dental Insurance Alternatives

Health maintenance organizations (HMOs) administer capitation programs, where the dentist gets a fixed fee based on the number of patients he/she serves. Medicare is an example of a contract fee schedule plan, in which dentists in the plan agree to accept defined, reduced fees for specific services. Managed care plans focus on preventive care and limit the procedures that can be performed or medications that can be prescribed. Direct reimbursement plans do not use an insurance carrier as an intermediary; here the patient pays for services and then is refunded money by his/her employer, who is the plan administrator.

Submitting Insurance Claims

Each completed dental procedure is assigned a five-digit CDT code that begins with a D for dental. CDT codes are described in the ADA's Current Dental Terminology. The patient must endorse on the claim form their assignment of benefits, which states that the benefits should be paid from the insurance carrier directly to the dentist or other provider. In lieu of an endorsement, there is a tacit agreement that the patient will pay for services independently. A signature on file can also be used for assignment of benefits. The patient signs another area for release of information to the carrier. The form has fields for patient identification. Insurance claims can be submitted by mail or electronically. Carriers have established schedules of benefits, detailing amounts they will reimburse for various activities.

Accounts Payable

Accounts Payable responsibilities are assigned to the bookkeeper or office manager. Some functions that require clinical knowledge, such as inventory supply and control, are assigned to the dental assistant. The total amount of Accounts Receivable (A/R) is the practice's gross income. Accounts Payable (A/P) is money paid out for various expenses. Deduct the A/P from the gross income to determine the net income or profit. Permanent salaries, mortgage payments, and utilities are steady fixed expenses. Monthly expenses that change, such as supplies or repairs, are variable expenses. The combination of fixed and variable expenses is the practice's overhead. Once or twice monthly, the dentist authorizes payment of Accounts Payable. There may be petty cash kept at Reception to cover incidental costs, like taxi couriers.

Supplies

The dental assistant usually orders supplies because he/she has clinical knowledge and surveys the stock daily. Supplies are either expendable (disposable and quickly consumed) or non-expendable (enduring and purchased rarely). The assistant must consider:
Shelf life (expiry date) and rate of use
Storage space and special requirements (e.g., ice, dark, dry, fume hood)
Single item price, unit price for grouped items, and bulk price (cut-rate price for

ordering a minimum number of units), and price break (the smallest number of units needed to obtain a bulk price)

Lead time between ordering and delivery, which determines the reorder point at which a supply needs to be bought in order to ensure continued availability

Two common methods of reordering supplies are the red flag reorder tag system and the electronic bar code system. In the red flag reorder tag system, a tag is affixed to an item in inventory at the previously identified reorder point. At minimum, the name of the supply is on the tag. When the product reaches the reorder point, the tag is removed and put in a specified area for reordering. Every type of supply has an index card with information needed for ordering. The tag is attached to the upper-right corner when the item should be ordered, the left-hand corner after ordering, and removed upon receipt. New inventory is placed in the back of the pile and the red tag reaffixed at the new reorder point. With an electronic bar code system, supplies that must be reordered are identified by a specific bar code that is kept in a book. The assistant sweeps a bar code wand over the appropriate code, inputs the number of items needed, and the order is sent directly to the supplier via computer.

Examine all supplies received for damage. Look for inaccuracies and backorders on the packing slip enclosed with the shipment. If there is any damage or discrepancies, contact the supplier. Regular suppliers do not enclose a statement of payment due; it is sent separately to the practice on a monthly basis. A backorder is an item not immediately available; the supplier gives an estimated shipment date. If any units are returned, the supplier should issue the practice a credit slip, indicating there will be no charge. After receipt, the dental assistant should transfer the supplies to a well-organized storage area. Place older items in front to be utilized first. In a dental office, certain items are stored in a refrigerator or in a dark, dry spot. Controlled substances must be in a locked cabinet.

Remember that thieves target dental offices for gold and addicts look for narcotics and syringes.

Lab Equipment Maintenance

All dental laboratory equipment must be decontaminated and maintained in safe condition or retired. A dental laboratory technician may perform maintenance of complex equipment at your office, but often it is the dental assistant's responsibility. Much of the equipment is for taking impressions, creating trays, or making casts. These include the gypsum vibrator, extruder guns, lathes, model trimmer, hydrocolloid conditioning unit, soldering and welding equipment, and vacuum former. Most of these ship with explicit manufacturer-provided instructions, or you can obtain a copy from the sales person. Instruments that must be cleaned between uses and checked for wear include spatulas, laboratory knives, reusable impression trays, flexible rubber bowls, and measuring devices.

Instrument Care

Most dental instruments are made of stainless steel, or occasionally aluminum or high-tech resins. Clean them promptly after use by immersion in an ultrasonic bath or instrument washer. Instruments that cannot be cleaned right away should be presoaked temporarily. Separate the blades of all instruments. Ultrasonic solution should cover all the instrument parts. Instruments that have hinges (e.g., scissors and forceps) should be sanitized first and later sterilized in the open position. Remove instruments from the ultrasonic bath, hold them under running water, dry, and then sterilize them. Sterilization techniques include liquid chemical disinfectants, ethylene oxide, hot glass bead, dry heat, chemical vapor, and steam autoclave sterilization. Dry the instruments well prior to storage. Some instruments have different or additional maintenance requirements. For example, burrs and handpieces must be scrubbed first,

and since handpieces are attached to a power
source via tubing, they need initial flushing
and lubrication.

Radiologic Imaging Concept/Process

Pioneer Wilhelm Conrad Roentgen

Wilhelm Conrad Roentgen is credited with being the discoverer of X-rays. In November 1895, as a physics professor at University of Wurzburg in Germany, he was performing experiments involving the flow of electric current in a vacuum tube. Even though the room was dark and the vacuum tube was covered with cardboard, fluorescent plates in the room glowed. Roentgen found that the intensity of the glowing was inversely related to the distance of the plate from the tube. He observed that the outline of the bones in his hand was weakly visible when he inadvertently put his hand between the plate and tube; he recorded similar observations of his wife's hand on a photographic plate. Roentgen named this previously unknown phenomenon "X-rays" because "x" is often used as the unknown in algebraic equations; others called the rays "roentgen rays" as a tribute to Roentgen and the field of study was termed roentgenology. Roentgen's work was verified within days by Thomas Alva Edison's laboratory in New Jersey.

Roentgen's dentistry work

In January 1896, a German dentist called Dr. Otto Walkhoff, made the first dental radiograph. He took a lower premolar X-ray by exposing himself to X-rays for 25 minutes while lying prone with an unexposed photographic plate in his mouth. In February 1896, physicist Walter Koenig made a clearer similar radiographic image with a shortened exposure time of 9 minutes. A New Orleans dentist called Dr. C. Edmond Kells demonstrated the use of X-rays to the Southern Dental Society in April 1896. The initial dental x-ray department was also set up that year by William Rollins. Most of these early researchers developed radiation burns or other side effects. The year 1913 heralded many other breakthroughs in the field of roentgenology including use of film instead of a photographic plate, invention of the hot-cathode x-ray tube, and introduction of the first American manufactured dental x-ray apparatus.

Atom structure

An atom is the smallest portion into which an element can be divided and still retain its inherent properties. Elements are the simplest units of matter and they cannot be broken down into other substances by chemical reactions. The number of identified elements has changed over time; 105 is the current number in 2007. The atom is comprised of a central nucleus containing a set number of positively charged protons and neutral neutrons which is surrounded by rings or orbits of negatively charged electrons. These electrons stay in orbit because of centrifugal force and their electrostatic attraction to the protons. The atomic or Z number is an expression of the number of protons or electrons in the atom.

Orbital electrons and binding energies

Electrons circle around the nucleus in up to 7 different paths or shells, which are sequentially lettered from K to Q. Shell K is closest to the nucleus, and shell Q is the theoretical furthest path. Normally, there is equilibrium between the centrifugal and electrostatic forces that enables each electron to stay in orbit. However, electrons in the outer orbital shells are more easily removed from the atom since less work or energy is required to strip the electrons from outer orbital shells than the inner paths. Electrons occupying the external shell are called valence electrons because they are easily removed and can thus establish the atom's chemical properties including its optical spectrum. Binding energy is the amount of energy needed to extract an electron from its orbit; this parameter is distinctive for each element and each orbital shell.

Electron volt and binding energy

An electron volt is a measurement of kinetic or motion-related energy. It is defined as the amount of energy generated by moving an electron through an electrical potential difference of 1 volt. It is often expressed as kiloelectron (keV) or megaelectron (MeV) volts, which are 1000 or 1 million times a single volt. Each shell of an atom has a defined binding energy which is generally expressed in keV. Electrons can be removed from the shell if that binding energy is achieved through bombardment with x-rays or other rays or particles. While loosely held electrons in the outermost paths can be removed by low energy visible light or UV rays, electrons in the closer shells can only be pulled off with higher energy x-rays, gamma rays, or certain particles.

Ionization and x-ray use

Ionization is the conversion of an atom from a neutral to either a positive or negative charge. The charge represents the discrepancy between the number of protons in the nucleus and the number of electrons after ionization, and the charged atom is called an ion. If outer orbital shells are unfilled, the atom has a tendency to acquire electrons, and it becomes a negatively charged anion. If electrons are lost, the result is a positively charged atom or cation. X-ray bombardment of an atom conveys energy to the orbital electron; the electron is ejected but forms a loose attraction to the atom termed an ion pair.

Particulate radiations

Particulate radiations are small masses that travel linearly at rapid speed and can penetrate matter. Only one type of particulate radiation is neutral in charge, the neutron. All of the other types are electrically charged, and the degree of penetration is generally inversely related to the particle mass. One variety is the alpha particle, the helium nucleus without the associated electrons, which is 2 protons plus 2 neutrons. These particles are emitted from heavy metals and are heavy and highly charged; thus alpha particles lose energy quickly and do not penetrate matter as well as other types of particulate radiation. The much smaller electrons penetrate tissue and air much more effectively. Electrons are emitted as particulate radiations as either beta particles (negatrons) from radioactive nuclei or as cathode rays (electrons). Cathode rays are actually flows of orbital electrons that are generated from the filament of an x-ray tube and travel from the cathode to the anode. The nuclei of the hydrogen atom can be speeded up and emitted as another form of particulate radiation, a proton, but the mass of these protons is large and they do not penetrate very effectively.

Electromagnetic radiation and diagnostic radiology

Electromagnetic radiation is energy traveling in space while generating electric and magnetic force fields. There are two types of electromagnetic radiation, gamma rays discharged from disintegrating radioactive nuclei, and x-rays emitted outside the nucleus without mass or electrical charge. X-rays can travel through tissues further than other forms of radiation without focal localization, making them important for forms of diagnostic radiology including dental radiographs. Particulate radiation like alpha and beta particles or the electromagnetic gamma rays are more useful in nuclear medicine treatments.

Electromagnetic radiation and wave propagation

Electromagnetic radiations, including X-rays, disseminate energy in wave-like patterns. The speed of dissemination of these rays is equivalent to the speed of light, which is defined as either 186,000 miles per second or

3×10^8 miles per second. Electromagnetic waves are distinguished by the fact that they do not require a medium to pass through; instead they can spread in a vacuum. X-rays and other waves are characterized by the interrelated constant speed of light (often shown as the letter c) and the variables of wavelength and frequency. Wavelength is the length between the same phase in adjoining waves, and it is usually expressed in meters or the Greek letter lambda. Frequency is the number of wave cycles occurring per second, it is measured in hertz, and it can be represented by the Greek letter nu. The relationship between these is: speed of light = wavelength (meters) x frequency (hertz or cycles/sec).

Electromagnetic radiation and additional particle concept

In addition to spreading in a wave-like pattern, x-rays and other narrow wavelength, high frequency electromagnetic radiations can act like particles. Distinct parcels of energy called quanta or photons are disseminated by these types of radiations. These energy bundles do not have mass. If the frequency of the wavelength is increased (in other words, the wavelength is shortened), the energy of the photon is increased proportionately. If the energy level reaches or exceeds 15 electron volts, orbital electrons of atoms can be pulled off. This is known as ionization and the associated types of rays are considered to be ionizing radiation; examples of this type of radiation include not only x-rays but gamma rays and certain types of ultraviolet rays.

Components of electromagnetic spectrum

The electromagnetic spectrum is the entire range of electromagnetic types of radiation. It is defined by the classification of the type of radiation and its associated wavelength range. The wavelength differences represented in the spectrum are quite large. The long wavelength, low frequency forms are alternating current, radio waves,

television, and radar; these wave cycles range from about 10^{12} meters down to several meters. Infrared, visible, and ultraviolet light have mid-range wavelengths. Ionizing radiations such as gamma rays and x-rays have extremely short wavelengths, and are thus often represented in nanometers (nm), or 10^{-9} meters. The effective wavelengths for medical or dental x-rays are about 0.01 to 0.05 nanometers. Another unit of measurement is the angstrom unit (A) or 1/10 of a nanometer.

Dentistry and medicinal characteristics of x-rays

X-rays are extremely short wavelength electromagnetic radiations that travel at the speed of light. They have no mass. They disseminate in wave-like patterns in a straight line, but they can be redirected into other linear paths. X-ray beams spread out with increasing distance from the source. X-rays can go through materials that are impenetrable by longer wavelength sources. Certain materials such as photographic film can selectively absorb x-rays. X-rays can trigger fluorescence, or the emission of longer wavelength radiation, in some substances, and this property is often exploited to amplify the response. X-rays can ionize substances including gases; this property is utilized in ionization chambers. X-rays can also induce changes in biological materials such as human tissues, and this is the basis for their utility in therapeutic radiology.

Simple x-ray tube setup

A simple x-ray tube consists of a tightly closed housing made of leaded glass (usually Pyrex), a negative terminal or cathode comprised of a tungsten filament wire surrounded by a molybdenum cup, and a positively charged copper anode with a central area made of tungsten. The tungsten filament of the cathode serves as a source of electrons when heated. These electrons are set in motion by the application of an extremely high voltage or electrical potential difference between the cathode and anode. The central area of the anode is called the focal spot; at the focal spot, about 1% of the energy generated is changed into x-rays with the remainder dissipated as heat production or infrared radiation in the outer portions of the anode. The anode serves as means of suddenly stopping or decelerating the electrons. Tungsten filaments are used because they have very high melting points and are destroyed.

Benson line focus and design of dental x-ray tubes

The path of x-rays can be deflected, and this property is exploited in the design of dental x-ray tubes to sharpen images. The Benson line focus principle reduces the effective dimensions of the focal spot. This is accomplished by an anode design with an angled face to the electron path, typically at 15 to 20 degrees relative to the cathode. When the electrons strike the focal spot, they are therefore deflected through an x-ray window below the diverted path to the photographic film. The resultant "effective" focal spot is considerably smaller than the spot on the anode and image quality is improved. In addition, the anode can absorb more heat because it is spread over a larger area of that electrode.

Electron generation in an x-ray tube

Electrons are generated in the tungsten filament of the cathode of the x-ray tube. When the filament is heated, thermal energy is transmitted to the tungsten and the electrons in its outer orbital shells are stripped off to form a cluster of electrons. This phenomenon is known as thermionic emission. Tungsten does not melt until it reaches 3370 degrees Centigrade, and the filament is typically heated to about two-thirds of that melting point. The rate of electron flow or electrical current measured in milliamperes (mA) is directly related to the applied temperature and the number of electrons pulled off. A typical dental x-ray apparatus generates between 7 and 15 milliamperes.

Function of the cathode focusing cup in an x-ray tube

The focusing cup is a receptacle that surrounds the tungsten filament of the x-ray tube cathode. It is usually made of molybdenum. The main purpose of the focusing cup is to direct the flow of electrons to the anode so that they strike a smaller, more focused area of the anode. Otherwise, the electron beam would spread out more, electrons would strike a larger portion of the anode, and the image would not be very distinct. The speed of electron flow is controlled by the amount of potential difference or voltage between the two electrodes. While there is a maximum voltage or peak (kVp or kilovoltage peak) that can be applied, the actual voltage of individual electrons is variable and usually less that the maximum A greater gap potential difference will produce a faster electron flow or current, and subsequently x-ray photons with higher frequencies and energies are generated. Higher energy x-rays can penetrate further than those with lower energies.

Electrons in x-ray tubes

Electrons streaming from the cathode to the anode in an x-ray tube have what is termed kinetic or motion-related energy. When these electrons reach the anode, they are stopped or decelerated. A portion of these electrons hit the tungsten target where the electrons in the shell orbits of the tungsten become excited. This means that these latter electrons temporarily possess higher energy levels, but as they revert to their initial states energy is given off in the form of either infrared radiation (heat) or as x-rays. The small proportion of x-rays generated (less than 1% usually) are redirected in many directions in the tube, and the x-rays that manage to pass through the x-ray window represent the useful beam for imaging and other purposes.

Bremsstrahlung radiation

In an x-ray tube, two types of radiation are produced, Bremsstrahlung (general radiation) and characteristic radiation. Bremsstrahlung (also called Brems or general radiation) is the dominant type of x-ray elicited by dental x-ray equipment. This general radiation represents photons of energy emitted as a result of a deceleration of the high-speed electrons at the tungsten anode target. This occurs in one of two ways. Usually, high-speed electrons streaming from the cathode are attracted to the positively charged nucleus of the tungsten in the anode target. If opposing nuclear forces are stronger, the fast electron is deflected and slowed down near the nucleus and x-ray photons are emitted. This pattern of attraction followed by deflection, deceleration, and photon emission continues until the electron's energy is depleted. On the other hand, if the high-speed electron actually collides with and penetrates the nucleus, only one discrete photon of x-ray energy is produced.

Characteristic radiation and a typical x-ray tube

Characteristic radiation is a type of x-ray that is generated when a high-energy electron from the cathode ionizes or removes an electron from an inner orbit of the target. A typical x-ray tube has a tungsten target at the anode. If the cathode electrons hit the target with enough energy, an electron in the innermost K shell of the tungsten is initially ejected. Subsequently, an electron from the next L shell moves to occupy the space in the K shell where the electron was pulled off, and a photon of so-called "characteristic radiation" is released. Characteristic radiation represents the disparity between the binding energies in the two orbital shells, and it is always the same for a particular element (tungsten in this case). In an x-ray tube, a photon of characteristic radiation is 59 keV, or the difference between the binding energy of the K shell of tungsten, 70 keV, and the L shell, 11 keV. This type of radiation is only emitted if the potential difference in the tube equals or exceeds the 70 keV binding energy of the K shell.

Heterogeneous vs. homogeneous

Most Brems radiation emitted from a typical dental x-ray tube controlled by alternating current (AC) is heterogeneous. This means that the radiation is released in a range of energies and wavelengths. This variety occurs for two reasons. First, the electrons coming from the cathode possess a continuum of speeds due to the AC, and second, most of the electrons gradually lose energy by a series of interactions with different nuclei. Longer wavelength photons either bounce around inside the tube or are filtered out. If the apparatus is designed to convert the AC to direct current (DC), then a more homogeneous radiation is effectively emitted, greater penetration of the soft tissues is achieved, and image quality is improved. This is because all the cathode-derived electrons achieve the same voltage difference near the peak applied, and the subsequent radiation emitted is more uniform as well. This also allows for somewhat lower doses of radiation because there are no relatively useless longer wavelength species.

Self-rectification of current

Most x-ray generators provide electrical energy to the dental x-ray tube in the form of alternating current (AC), typically as 110 or 220 volts in cycles of 60 Hertz (Hz or cycles per second). This means that the electrons generated flow first in one direction from the cathode to the anode by attraction, and then in the other direction. A wavelike pattern is produced in which the current reaches a peak, returns to baseline, and then goes through a trough and return to baseline when the current is reversed. During this latter trough, current does not stream through the x-ray tube because the anode is already negatively charged. The result is self-rectification or effective conversion of the alternating current to unidirectional direct current (DC). In addition, while direction of the AC is changed every 1/120 of a second, the number of useful cycles per second is halved (in other words, 60 Hz).

Typical x-ray generator

A typical x-ray generator used for dental x-rays is comprised of two distinct parts. The first is the control panel which contains all of the controls for parameters such as the exposure time, current selection (mA or milliamperes), potential difference (kVp or kilovoltage peak), and the like plus the actual x-ray emission light. The other part is the tubehead assembly which consists of the x-ray tube and transformers. All of the tubehead assembly is submerged in oil to shield the apparatus and thwart sparks between different components.

Utilizing Transformers

Transformers are electromagnetic pieces of equipment that step the voltage potential difference up or down in an efficient manner. They usually consist of an iron core surrounded by two different loops of wire at either end. As the current passes through the core and the first or primary circuit wire, a magnetic field is generated. This in turn sets up a secondary current in the second loop of wire if the magnitude of the magnetic field is shifting such as when alternating current is applied. The number of times each wire is coiled around the end relative to the other wire determines whether the transformers can step-up or step-down the voltage. The voltage generated in the secondary coil is directly related to the number of coils it possesses relative to the primary wire loop. Some dental x-ray machines have variable autotransformers in which there is only one large coil encircling the iron core. In this case, there are multiple areas where the insulation of the wire has been removed; a metal conductor can be moved to different

exposed areas to generate and control the magnitude of the secondary circuit.

Transformers changes in dental x-ray machines

In a dental x-ray machine, a filament circuit is activated when the exposure switch is closed. When a step-down transformer is used, the voltage is decreased from the applied 110 or 220 volts in the primary loop to a much lower voltage of about 8 to 12 volts in the secondary wire. This generates a large current of about 3 to 6 amperes to heat the cathode filament which in turn produces more electrons there. If a step-up transformer is utilized instead, the applied current is increased in the secondary coil to a very high voltage of about 60 to 100 kVp. In this case, this extreme potential difference accelerates the movement of the cathode electrons to the anode, while also decreasing the current to about 10 to 15 milliamperes. Autotransformers are typically used as step-up transformers that can vary the voltage.

X-ray beam intensity

The intensity of an x-ray beam is its total energy emitted per unit area and time. Total energy is the product of two key components, the quantity or number of photons in the beam and the quality or energy of the specific photons. Area is defined in terms of the cross-sectional space at the point of measurement on the film; this is proportional to the distance from the source which can be controlled. The exposure rate or time can also be regulated by the technician as can the voltage and current applied. Thus the beam intensity can be calculated as:

Intensity = (quantity of photons x quality)/(cross-sectional area x exposure time)

- 99 -

X-ray emission spectrum and the current applied

The current applied using a dental x-ray apparatus is directly related to the number of electrons produced at the cathode filament and the subsequent number of electrons flowing to the electrode. For each heterogeneous x-ray beam, there is a spectrum of emission of x-rays of various wavelengths or photons of different energies. This can be represented in a distribution curve. The setup of a particular machine can shift the proportion of types of x-rays emitted, but in general the beam intensity can be proportionately affected by changes in the current (mA) applied and the electron flow.

Exposure time and current

More photons of x-ray energy are generated by increasing the exposure time. Often the maximum potential difference (kVp) and current (mA) are preset when doing dental x-rays, and the only variable is the exposure time. In this case, increasing exposure time augments the total energy or intensity. Exposure time can be expressed as either fractions or whole multiples of a second or as the number of impulses of electrical energy applied in a second. Either expression of exposure time can be multiplied by the current applied to give values known as mAs or mAi respectively. In general, the goal is to maintain either mAs or mAi as constant, which can be achieved by changing the current and exposure time in opposition. In other words, if the current is increased the exposure time is decreased and vice versa.

X-ray tube potential difference

The kilovoltage or potential difference applied influences the number and degree of penetration of the x-rays emitted. Potential differences of between 60 and 65 kVp generate x-rays that do not penetrate much and are termed "soft"; these x-rays have relatively long wavelengths and low frequencies and energies. Larger potential differences of usually 85 to 100 kVp produce x-rays that penetrate either much more or completely and are termed "hard". Here the associated x-ray wavelengths are relatively short, and the energies and frequencies are higher. These differences can be exploited when performing dental x-rays by using larger voltages in areas that are thick or dense.

Voltage changes

When voltage is increased, the intensity of the emitted x-ray increases as well. However, this relationship is more than linear; the factor the voltage is stepped up by must be squared to calculate the intensity. In addition, voltage increases are related to the current produced and ideal exposure time. A particular density or darkness of the film is usually desired. To achieve this density, there are two schemes generally followed. One states that the current in milliamperes should be cut in half for every 15% augmentation in voltage. Alternatively, the exposure time must be divided in two for every voltage rise of 15 kVp or doubled for each similar reduction of potential difference.

Inverse square law and positioning devices

X-rays generated at the target on the anode are filtered through a collimating device upon leaving the tube head. Then these rays are usually directed to the patient through the use of a beam- or position-indicating device. The intensity of the x-ray beam at the film in the patient's mouth is related to the distance of the film from the target source by a relationship called the inverse square law. This law states that the intensity of the radiation at the level of the film is inversely related to the square of the distance between the source and the film. For example, doubling the length of the positioning device cuts down the radiation intensity on the film by a factor of 4 (in other words, $2^2 = 4$). This can be compensated for by increasing the exposure time by the same factor of 4.

Film fog causes

Film fog or undesired darkness occurs when radiation that has been scattered touches the film. There are two ways in which these changes of direction can occur. A small portion of the radiation can undergo Thompson scattering, also known as unmodified or coherent scattering. In this case, lower energy photons change direction when they encounter matter but little else occurs. Another phenomenon called Compton or incoherent is more prevalent and it is a potentially greater problem for x-ray interpretation. Here higher energy x-rays expel outermost orbital electrons upon interaction with matter; this results in a positively charged atom loosely coupled to a negatively charged Compton or recoil electron. The origin photon changes direction and undergoes subsequent similar interactions and directional changes. If the angle of change is small, most of the intensity of the photon remains and it can easily arrive at the film as fog. The majority of dental x-ray photons experience this type of scattering so manipulations are usually necessary to reduce it. These manipulations can include use of rectangular collimators and changing other parameters to shorten exposure time.

Interactions that can occur

X-rays can be taken into matter and tissues when the two interact, a process called photoelectric absorption. This generally happens when the energy level of the photon is slightly greater than the binding energy of the material's K or innermost orbital shell. The x-ray is absorbed into and transfers its energy to the orbital electron which is expelled and taken in by another atom. Atoms with higher atomic numbers tend to absorb x-rays more readily. Photoelectric absorption is more prevalent with high frequency, low wavelength x-rays or when the interacting material is thick or dense. This phenomenon has also been classified as characteristic radiation; the energies to expel the K shell electron and replace it with an L

shell electron are both predetermined. The energy difference defines the energy of the resultant x-ray. A small portion of x-rays go right through the tissues without contact, but remnants from this type of interaction can still be seen as dark film spots after processing.

Different structures on film

Tissues and other materials found in the jaw area are subject to differential absorption of x-rays. Metals used in restorations tend to have high atomic numbers and thus absorb a greater proportion of x-rays. Therefore, restorations and to a lesser extent enamel and cortical bone usually are observed on x-ray films as radiopaque areas. This means that those areas are very bright and transparent because they have already absorbed the x-ray energy and it does not strike the film. At the other end of the spectrum, dark or radiolucent portions of the radiograph result from areas that are easily penetrated by the x-ray. These include the softer tissues. Scattering can produce similar dark spots. Teeth and bones are comprised of a considerable amount of calcium and phosphorus, which both have mid-range atomic numbers (20 and 15), but the rate of absorption can be affected by age and presence of decay or other disease in these structures.

Radiographic film composition

Typical radiographic film is double-sided or double-emulsion film. In the center of the film, there is a transparent, blue-colored plastic sheet or base. An emulsion is attached to either side of the base with some type of adhesive. The emulsion is a mixture of silver halide or silver iodo-bromide crystals, which interact with x-ray photons to produce what is known as a latent or invisible image, and clear gelatin. The silver compounds usually employed are 90% or greater silver bromide (chemical formula $AgBr$) and silver iodide (AgI) as the remainder. The outer layer on both sides of the radiographic film is a protective coating.

Latent image

Before the addition of developer, an invisible or latent image is produced in the radiographic emulsion. The silver, bromine and iodine atoms typically present in an emulsion form crystals that are bound by the electrovalence forces of ionic bonding. When x-rays bombard these crystals, they eject energetic photoelectrons and a chain reaction is set up. When these released electrons encounter deliberately manufactured imperfections or specks of silver sulfide, the electrons are trapped in that position. A cascade of positively charged silver ions is then attracted to the trapped electrons, and silver atoms are produced to form what is known as a latent or invisible image. When development chemicals are added, the silver catalyzes the reaction that makes these images visible.

Extraoral and intraoral dental x-ray films

Extraoral x-ray films (screen films) are indirectly exposed by changing the x-ray photons to light energy by use of screens on either side of the film. In the process, the signal is also amplified facilitating a smaller dosage of radiation. This technique is useful for documenting larger areas. Light sensitive films are used. Intraoral films directly expose the radiation to the film. These types of films are used only for small areas inside the oral cavity. They come as separately enclosed double-emulsion films protected by a lead backing which provides stiffness, protects against further scattering, and catches excess radiation. Current films of this type always identify the side to be placed against the x-ray tube with a raised dot.

Types and sizes of intraoral x-ray films

Intraoral x-ray films can be described in terms of type or area of documentation. There are three types. The first, the periapical film, is used to record the apical or top area of the tooth, nearby bone structures and crown. This type of film comes in a single child size (No. 0) and two adult sizes (No. 1 for the front and No. 2 for the back and bitewings as well). Bitewing films are used to simultaneously document the crown area and the interproximal alveolar bone crests. This can be accomplished by added a tab to the No. 2 film above, using some type of holder, or combining use of two films. Occlusal films (size 3) are much bigger and are designed for use in larger areas like the floor of the mouth. Other numbering systems have child (#0), narrow frontal (#1), adult (#2), preformed bitewing (#3) and occlusal (#4) sizes available.

Intraoral films size and speed

The American Dental Association has classified intraoral films by a number that combines both the type and size of the film. Periapical film classifications are generically represented by 1.x where x is the size of the film. Similarly, bitewing films are defined as 2.x, with x again being the size. There is one type of standard occlusal film, the 3.4. Radiographic film speed is really a reflection of the sensitivity of the film. High speed x-ray films generate radiographic images with relatively short exposure times. Currently there are three speeds of film available, the fastest group F and slower groups E and D, but in theory the slowest film speed would be classified as group A. The fastest speed films have been achieved in recent years by the Eastman Kodak Company by incorporation of tabular shaped (instead of round) grains into the emulsion, thus increasing effective surface area.

Handling dental x-ray films

Closed boxes of dental x-ray film need to be kept in a refrigerator or other cool area. After opening, the unused film should either be stowed in lead containers or away from the screening area (intraoral) or near the area but in containers that block light (screen film). This is because the emulsions are responsive to a number of situations including excessive heat, light exposure, other radiation, touching, and gas fumes. Films designed for use at high speeds are more finely tuned and thus even more susceptible to these factors.

Diagnostic quality

The diagnostic or radiographic quality of a dental radiograph is the exactitude of the representation of anatomical structures and their clarity on the film. This clarity is comprised of the sharpness or definition of the various structures on the film plus the detail or micro-architecture of these structures. Quality radiographs should demonstrate the proper density and contrast, they should be anatomically correct, they should include all areas of interest, and they need to be sharp. Sharpness or definition can be improved by minimizing distortion and various inherent impediments as well as by controlling magnification.

Measuring radiographic density

Radiographic films are interpreted by observing them facing an illuminator or view-box. Radiographic density is a measurement of the amount of light that passes through a radiographic film relative to the intensity of the light striking it from behind the illuminator. The density is a reading of the relative darkness, blackness, or radiolucency of areas of the film. The parameter is a reflection of the composition of the film, variables employed during the radiation procedure, and the size of the resultant silver aggregates. Density is defined by a logarithmic relationship as the $\log_{10}$ of the proportion between the intensity of incident light (I) and that transmitted through the film (T). This translates to a density of 1.0 if 1/10 of the light passes through and a density of 2.0 if 1/100 is transmitted, which are radiographic densities usually considered acceptable versus very dark. Technicians sometimes use densities as light as 0.3.

Variables that affect density

Aspects of the actual radiographic exposure are the most important variables that control radiographic density, particularly the product mAs. Milliampere seconds, or mAs, is the multiplication product between the current in milliamperes times the exposure time in seconds; it is important because it directly affects the number of x-rays hitting the film and the amount of silver that aggregates. The kilovoltage difference in the x-ray tube is also significant because it controls the wavelength and frequency of the x-rays, and the most penetrating x-rays occur with high voltage and resultant short wavelengths. Density is also inversely related to the square of the distance between the x-ray beam and the film. There are other less important factors that contribute to the control of radiographic density including film speed, use of grid devices to filter out scattering, and utilization of screens that change x-ray into light energy. During the development process, it is also possible to under develop the film if chemicals are depleted.

Long-scale vs. short-scale contrast

Radiographic contrast is the difference between the densities of extremely dark and light portions of a radiograph. The most important factor controlling contrast is the kilovoltage potential difference in the x-ray tube. Generally, at lower kilovoltages of 60 to 65 kV, short-scale contrast is observed; at these voltages, the x-rays emitted have long wavelengths but lower energy. Since relatively few silver aggregates are formed on the film, there are not many gradations between light and dark in the image. On the other hand, if higher voltages of 80 to 90 kV are used, long-scale contrast is usually observed. Here the x-rays have shorter wavelengths and greater penetrability, and more silver bundles develop resulting in more gradations of gray. An aluminum step wedge device, also called a penetrometer, can be used to measure these changes.

Recommendation of long- or short-scale radiographic contrast

Use of long-scale radiographic contrast conditions is generally preferred for radiographs of the periapical areas and bony changes like periodontal or periapical disease. Conditions favoring short-scale radiographic contrast are usually recommended for bitewing images and the illustration of caries or tooth decay. Ideal densities and contrasts are subjective, however. Low voltage, short-scale films, may not show early pathologic alterations. Long-scale films with their gradations can identify early changes better, and some clinicians prefer these for caries. The downside of long-scale films is that they are not as crisp and visually pleasing.

Exposure time relationships

Is theoretically controlled by the kilovoltage applied. The density or darkness of a film is affected by a number of factors; the most important variable is milliampere seconds but kilovoltage also increases the density. When either exposure time or the mAs product is altered, film density is changed but contrast is not unless the kVp potential difference is also changed. In practice, lower mAs (and exposure times) are usually utilized with the higher voltages producing low or long-scale contrast, and higher values of these parameters are generally used with lower voltages and high or short-scale contrast.

Characteristic curve and contrast

A characteristic curve is a xy plot of film density (y) versus the logarithm of the exposure time (x). Each type of film has its own characteristic curve. The plot looks like an elongated S with a bottom or toe part, a long relatively straight line portion in the middle, and a shoulder at the top. The middle straight line part of the curve can be defined by its slope, or the change in the density relative to log of relative exposure time (y/x).

The straight line portion is also the zone of correct exposure. Films with steeper slopes provide more contrast than those with shallower slopes.

Characteristic curve and acceptable exposure times relationships

The range of acceptable exposure times can also be extrapolated from the characteristic curve by drawing lines from the y density axis in the desired range (for example about 0.5 to 2.5); only exposure times falling in that range are diagnostically useful. There is a degree of tolerance or exposure error, termed latitude, inherent in the film that is inversely proportional to its slope and corresponding contrast. In other words, there is little latitude or room for error with high contrast films and vice versa. Kilovoltage applied affects the amount of latitude in the acceptable range of exposure times directly because of its inverse relationship to contrast.

Spatial characteristics

The central sharp area of a radiographic image is called the umbra, and it is surrounded by a blurrier area called the penumbra. The less sharp penumbra area can be reduced by decreasing the target area on the anode and the effective focal area. Images are also distorted on radiographs because materials furthest from the film will be magnified more than those closer. This distortion can influence the perceived shape of the tooth or other object as well. These distortions are related to the attempt to visualize three-dimensional objects on the flat plane of a film. Detail or definition is also influenced by the distances between the film and either the focal point or the object. Movement of the patient or any equipment or the use of intensifying screens can decrease definition and produce blurriness. Definition is directly related to contrast.

Geometric unsharpness and distortion

Geometric unsharpness or the amount of penumbra on the image is best controlled by

- 104 -

the use of an x-ray machine with a small focal spot on the anode target. This is an inherent property of the equipment and cannot be changed. As the distance between the focal spot and the film is increased, the sharpness increases. Conversely, as the distance between the object being documented and the film is increased, the sharpness decreases and more of the film is blurry. These distances primarily affect the magnification of certain areas and their relative distortion. The relationship between true object size and these parameters is as follows:

object size = (distance between source and object x length of image)/distance between x-ray source and film.

Minimizing radiographic distortion
Distortion caused by differences in shape and size can be minimized by two techniques, paralleling and bisecting. Paralleling refers to the placement of the long axis of the object in parallel to the film. Bisecting means positioning the radiation beam perpendicular to the midpoint of the angle between the film and the long axes of the teeth. Less distortion and greater anatomical accuracy is generally seen with the paralleling technique. In the bisecting technique, the depth dimension differs for various teeth and this can foreshorten or elongate the image.

Technique used to minimize distortion
The length of beam indicating (BID) or positioning device should be selected based on the technique employed to minimize distortion. The bisecting technique can only be performed with the shorter 8-inch BID generally; it allows the film to be positioned close to the teeth to be x-rayed. Any length device can be used for the paralleling technique since it is placed perpendicular to both the teeth and film. The longer tubes (16 inches generally) are better because the distance between focal space and object is increased and sharpness is subsequently augmented.

Assuring proper coverage

An x-ray should generally include visualization of five tissue types, the tooth enamel, its underlying dentin or hard calcium-containing portion, the sensitive central pulp with nerves and blood vessels, the alveolar or jaw bone, and the surrounding soft tissue. For a periapical film, several millimeters of bone should be seen. All areas needed for diagnostic purposes should be included if possible with the initial film or visualized on supplemental images such as occlusal films. There are also guidelines for inclusion of other areas like the periodontal membrane space and superimposition of certain cusp tips. Proper coverage can be attained by a combination of the accurate alignment of film and radiation beam, use of the correct film type, and amplification if necessary.

Radiation Health

Effects of x-radiation on atoms and molecules

When an x-ray photon comes in contact with an atom or molecule, the molecular structure is changed. In some cases, the energy from the photon causes orbital electrons in the atom to vibrate or become excited. The result is either release of light and heat or the actual disruption of molecular bonds. If the energy of the x-ray is enough to expel the orbital electron from the atom, a second phenomenon called ionization occurs. In this case, an electron can be ejected or loosely bound to form an ion pair with the now positively charged atom. If molecular bonds are broken, molecules act differently and cell function can be disrupted.

Radiolysis

Radiolysis is the breakdown of chemicals into smaller components by x-rays or other radiation. The term usually refers to the interface of this radiation with water molecules because water makes up about 4/5 of the body. Subsequently, an ion pair of the positively charged water and a free electron or radical is created. The term free radical can describe any molecule containing an unpaired electron, though, and all of these are very chemically reactive and able to destroy life components like deoxyribonucleic acid (DNA) and adenosine triphosphate (ATP). For example, two hydroxyl (OH-) radicals can combine to form a harmful substance called hydrogen peroxide (H_2O_2).

Radiation effects on biological materials

Radiation can affect biological materials either directly or indirectly. When radiation interacts directly with biologically active materials, the destruction is a direct effect. The most significant direct effect is the breakdown of DNA in the nucleus of the cell, which prevents further cell processes including replication resulting in cell death. Radiation can have a direct destructive effect on other important molecules like proteins and ribonucleic acid (RNA) as well. Ionizing radiation can also act indirectly by producing free radicals that later either react with life-sustaining molecules or form intermediate toxic substances that affect biological materials. The effects of radiation can be cell damage or in rare instances malignant changes.

Accumulative effect of radiation

It has been theorized that the biological effects of radiation are cumulative. That means that the untoward effects of radiation exposure accumulate in increments with each contact. The consensus opinion is also that low-dose ionizing radiation (like that used in dentistry) has a non-threshold, linear type of dose-response curve. The concept of accumulative effect is premised upon the idea that repair after radiation exposure is never complete. This cumulative effect eventually can lead to malignancies, birth defects, aging, and other diseases. Damaging effects are not evident until a certain amount of time, called the latent period, has elapsed between exposure and documented consequences. The potential effects of the radiation are dependent on a number of host factors and radiation parameters.

Areas of the body to avoid

Genetic abnormalities and malignancies can result from radiation exposure. For dental radiography, this dictates shielding the gonads and reproductive systems of patients to prevent these abnormalities or fetal congenital defects. Exposure to the bone marrow, thyroid gland, or unnecessary areas of skin should be avoided as well because of the possibility of development of leukemia or other malignancies. In addition, cataract development has been associated with exposure of the lens of the eye to radiation so that area should be avoided as well.

X-radiation of dental radiography

There are various types of radiation. The radiation from dental x-rays is sparsely ionizing. This means that the energy they transfer is dispersed and these x-rays are said to have a low linear energy transfer (LET). Other types of radiation, in particular alpha particles, have a higher LET, deposit the energy in more discrete bundles, and have a considerably higher potential for biological damage. In addition, very small quantities of radiation are used for dental radiographs, most of the x-rays do not reach internal tissues because they are absorbed by outer layers of the skin, and only small areas of the head and neck are generally exposed. Short but intense acute exposure to radiation is generally more damaging than prolonged but smaller chronic exposure. Dental radiography might be considered chronic exposure because of its low level, repetitive nature.

Radiation effects on certain people

Most mammals including humans are more susceptible to the effects of radiation than other species. It is difficult to pinpoint why certain Individual human beings are more sensitive to radiation damage than others. However, it has been demonstrated that certain human organs and tissues are more radiosensitive than others. The most sensitive cell types are those that divide very rapidly, in particular tissues involved with blood formation (like bone marrow) or reproduction (such as the ovary) or those cells that are already malignant; cells in these categories are killed relatively easily by exposure to radiation. The least sensitive cell types, termed radioresistant cells, are those that do not divide often such as muscle and nerve cells.

Effects of radiation transmitted to the next generation

In general, the changes induced by radiation exposure are only transmitted to the next generation when these effects occur in genetic or reproductive tissues. In these types of tissues, the radiation actually causes changes in the genetic material, and these changes are then passed on to the next generation. On the other hand, all other cell types are termed somatic; they include skin, connective tissues, nerves and a wide variety of other tissues and organs. When somatic tissues are changed by radiation exposure, these changes are not transmitted to the progeny.

Responses to radiation doses in somatic and genetic tissues

When somatic tissues are exposed to radiation, changes do not occur until a particular threshold radiation dose is reached. The relationship between the radiation dose and subsequent tissue damage is not linear, but looks like a curve on a two-dimensional plot. These effects do not affect the genetic makeup of the individual. Rather they include effects like sunburn or other skin reddening, hair loss, development of cataracts on the eye, or sterility. On the other hand, genetic changes such as those occurring in reproductive tissues involve mutations in the DNA that can be passed on to the next generation or cause malignancies. In these tissues, the relationship between the amount of radiation exposure and number of mutations is linear. These genetic tissues do not need a threshold dose of radiation before mutations occur (termed non-threshold). There are other cellular mechanisms that can moderate the effects of radiation such as repair of DNA and other structures, destruction of the cell by other cells called phagocytes, and stimulation of the immune system.

Measurement systems for radiation dose

The traditional units of measurement for radiation dose were the roentgen or R, rad and rem; all of these terms are equivalent and they are often expressed as 1/1000 or milliroentgens (mR), millirads (mrad), or millirems (mrem). While these units are still often used, there is also a newer SI classification system. In the SI system, units are expressed in gray (Gy) or sievert (Sv) units as well as 1/100 (centigray or cGy) and 1/1000 (milligray or mGy). The relationship between the two systems is 1 gray per 100 rads. These are all units of dose, or the amount of energy from the x-ray that is taken in per mass unit of tissue. For example, the gray unit represents the number of Joules of energy absorbed per kilogram of tissue. Dose absorbed is a more important parameter than exposure because it corresponds to potential biological destruction.

Radiation exposure vs. dose

Radiation exposure represents the number of photons producing a particular electrical charge in a volume of air. Originally, exposure was measured by converting the number of roentgen units, which quantified the number of ion pairs per cubic centimeter of air, into the electrical charge produced, which was expressed in coulombs or C. Today, exposure is expressed in exposure units, which are defined as one coulomb per kilogram of air. Exposure does not necessarily reflect the actual radiation dose delivered to tissues, and this dosage is highly dependent on a number of factors like tissue density and host response. The modern dose unit is the SI unit or gray. Dose was previously (and still is sometimes) expressed in rad; 1 rad is equivalent to 100 erg (a measurement of energy as well) absorbed per gram of tissue.

Dose equivalents

Different types of radiation can produce varying amounts of biological damage with the same dose. X-rays, beta particles, and gamma rays all possess the least potential for destruction. They have been assigned a quality factor (QF) of 1. Other more damaging types of radiation have been assigned higher QFs, which represent their relative destructive power. The concept of dose equivalents (H) expresses the relative destructive effects of different radiation types in sieverts or mSv by multiplying the dose (D) in Gy by the assigned quality factor (QF). All types of radiation (including x-rays) with a QF of 1 have equal doses and dose equivalents so the number of Gy and Sv are the same. For more destructive types of radiation like neutrons or alpha particles, the number of dose equivalents (Sv) is larger than the dose absorbed by a factor, the QF.

Effective dose equivalents

The risk of development of genetic defects or cancer from radiation exposure is dependent on the location and breadth of exposure in addition to the number of dose equivalents absorbed. The reason is that certain tissues are more susceptible to damaging biological effects and malignancy, in particular reproductive and blood-forming tissues and certain organs like the breast. Therefore, the concept of effective dose equivalents, or H(E) expressed in Sv or fractions thereof, defines the relative destructive power based on area of exposure. In dentistry for example, a bitewing or panoramic radiograph exposes the patient to very low effective dose equivalents, while a full-mouth intraoral set using multiple exposures and films multiplies this effective dose. Use of faster films lessens the effective dose. X-rays used in other settings such as nuclear medicine expose the patient to beams in much larger areas of the body including potential genetic targets and deliver much higher effective doses. They are often termed whole body exposures.

Greatest biological risks

The greatest biological risks from dental radiation exposure are the possible development of two types of malignancies, leukemia and thyroid cancer. Dental x-rays augment the natural probability that an individual may develop these cancers by increased exposure. Leukemia is cancer of the bone marrow, which is involved in blood cell production. Since about 10% of the body's bone marrow is in the skull region, and about a tenth of that is located in the actual mandible, dental radiography does slightly increase the probability of leukemia. The thyroid gland, the endocrine gland at the base of the neck, is close enough to the region typically irradiated during dental x-rays to be subject to scatter radiation. There are thyroid collars that can be worn by the patient to eliminate about half of the already low dose of scatter radiation.

Biological risks to other areas of the body are minimal with x-rays

Most dental offices utilize leaded torso aprons for their patients while taking dental x-rays, thus virtually eliminating whole body and specifically reproductive organ exposure. These aprons are especially important as preventive measures for pregnant females to reduce the possibility of fetal congenital defects. There are few documented studies about the effects of radiation on genetic changes in reproductive organs and subsequent transmission to children. Even without aprons, the uterus and fetus receive only minor secondary radiation. Other possible risks like cataract development require a threshold dose of radiation before untoward effects are observed. At the exposure levels of typical dental x-rays, the risk is very small because the values are far below the threshold.

Radiation caries

Radiation caries is the progressive decay of teeth or bones in the maxillofacial region after high dose radiation treatment of head or neck cancer. When doses of about 6000 rad are used to kill cancerous cells in the region, the softer tissues like the salivary glands are often affected as well. The amount of saliva produced is depleted and it becomes thicker. Friction in the mouth and the predilection towards development of caries are both increased. Another condition called osteoradionecrosis, or destruction of bone tissue, may also develop.

Sources of background radiation

The environment exposes individuals to background radiation. In the United States, this background level is about 3 mSv with the major type of exposure being from radon gas. In some other countries, the background radiation levels have been documented to be up to 13 times higher than in the United States without demonstrable changes in the population rate of malignancies or birth defects. Areas of high altitude have a slightly higher background level of radiation. Typically, the effective dose of ionizing radiation that an individual in the U. S. receives from dental x-rays is only about 0.1 percent of their total radiation received. Medical diagnostic procedures on average account for much greater doses experienced than dental x-rays. Nevertheless, background radiation undoubtedly supplies the greatest dosage, more than 4/5 of the total in the U. S. Total dosage in the U. S. is projected to be about 4.4 mSv per person.

Regulation bodies in the United States

There a number of bodies in the United States and internationally that make recommendations or actually govern radiation health and safety. In the United States, a subsidiary of the Food and Drug Administration (FDA), the National Center for Devices and Radiological Health (NCDRH) controls the manufacture of x-ray machines and other devices emitting radiation. Occupational exposure guidelines are established by the Nuclear Regulatory Commission (NRC), the Occupational Safety and Health Administration (OSHA), or indirectly by the Environmental Protection Agency (EPA) as well. There are also several nationally-based organizations that make recommendations related to radiation health and safety including the Biological Effects of Ionizing Radiation Committee (BEIR) operating under the National Academy of Sciences and the National Council on Radiological Protection and Measurement (NCRPM). Every state has a Bureau of Radiation Safety that regulates radiation procedures locally.

International organizations

Several international organizations keep abreast of radiation biology research and make recommendations based on current information. These bodies include the United Nations Scientific Committee on the Effects of Atomic Radiation (UNSCEAR) and the International Commission of Radiological Protection (ICRP). There is also an official world-wide group that proposes standards for radiological units of measurement called the International Commission on Radiation Units and Measurements (ICRU).

Determining MPD

MPD is the abbreviation for maximum permissible dose of radiation a person is permitted to receive from artificial causes of radiation. The MPD is generally a recommendation of the NCRPM which acquires legal status through local or federal legislation. The MPD is generally higher for groups that are occupationally exposed like dentists and their assistants than for staff members or the general public, who are said to be non-occupationally exposed. A radiation worker who is pregnant is allowed to receive approximately the same lower level of dosage permitted for those non-occupationally exposed. These limits are not imposed for dental or medical procedures that may utilize radiation for patient benefit.

Maximum permissible doses currently recommended in different categories
At present, the annual effective MPD dose for radiation workers is a whole body dose of 50 mSv, with higher amounts to certain body parts up to 750 mSv on the hands. Workers falling into this category are permitted to receive a cumulative lifetime exposure of 10 times their age in years (for example, 500 mSv for an individual 50 years of age). The public or anyone non-occupationally exposed should receive only 1or 5 mSv, depending on whether their exposure is continuous (as in several dental x-rays) or infrequent; doses to specific areas like the lens of the eye can approach 50 mSv. Anyone training in the dental profession who is younger than 18 years old is subject to these limits as well. A pregnant woman should never receive more than 0.5 mSv a month up to a maximum of 5 mSv during the time she carries the child. In practice, the recommendation is to permit "as low as reasonably achievable" (ALARA) radiation, which is hopefully lower than imposed MPD.

Lowering radiation dosage

This shift can be achieved either by using the higher 70 to 90 kVp potential difference in the tube, and/or filtering out the longer wavelength x-rays. The filtration is commonly accomplished by insertion of an aluminum filter. Legislation also dictates that the cross-sectional area of the beam can be no greater than 7 centimeters in diameter if round. Therefore, x-ray machines usually have diaphragms or collimators that restrict the beam area; rectangular is superior to round collimation because it lessens the exposed area, reduces scatter-induced fogging, and thus produces a better image as well. Selection of a longer 16 inch beam indicating device that is lined with lead restricts radiation dosage most effectively. Use of machines with integrated electronic timers provides more precision. In addition, some newer machines have generators that can convert AC to DC and thus produce a constant wavelength beam.

Reducing radiation to the patient outside the actual x-ray machine

Potential whole-body and thyroid irradiation can be drastically reduced through the use of leaded torso aprons and thyroid shields. Film selection is important because faster films allow for lower exposure times and less potential radiation dosage; the fastest is speed F. Gadgets that hold the film in place should be used for many reasons including elimination of finger exposure and more precise placement of the film relative to the teeth and the positioning device. For panoramic or extra oral films, special films that incorporate rare earth intensifying screens are available that augment film speed further.

Reduce radiation dosage through good darkroom and viewing techniques

Utilization of a variety of practices to ensure the proper development of radiographs eliminates the need for repeat x-rays and exposure to the patient. The potential for film fog should be reduced by careful measures to eliminate light leaks into the darkroom. Low 15 watt bulbs with appropriate safelight filters placed at least 4 feet from the development area should be used. Manual development should not be assessed visually; it should always continue for at least 5 minutes at 70°F. Quality control measures regarding the processing solutions should be in place. These measures should include periodic stirring and changing of the solution, especially if contamination has occurred. The chemical tray should be covered to avoid oxidation during periods of non-use and regularly cleaned. Elevated temperatures should be avoided as well. The radiographs should be viewed in a lowly lit room through an opaque view box.

ADA guidelines for taking radiographs

Exposure to radiation through use of dental radiographs is a clinical judgment call and it is not always necessary every dental visit. All radiographic exams should be individualized for new patients. Children who do not have permanent teeth yet may not require x-rays, but if the dentist cannot inspect certain areas of the mouth, some periapical, occlusal or posterior bitewing views might be taken. After their permanent teeth begin to erupt, these types of radiographs plus panoramic views are usually taken. For adolescents or adults with complete or at least partial dentition, posterior bitewings plus panoramic and/or some periapical views are typically done. If history or evidence of dental disease is present, a full mouth radiograph is usually taken. The diagnostic plan for edentulous or toothless adults should be very individualized based on clinical criteria.

ADA guidelines for use of radiographs for returning patients

The dentist should exercise clinical judgment before radiographs are done on returning patients. If the patient had previous caries or appears to be at risk for development of decay, then posterior bitewing radiographs are usually indicated at 6 to 12 month intervals for children or adolescents or up to 18 months for adults. If caries development or predilection was not previously observed, the period between bitewing x-rays can be increased up to 2 years for children and 3 years for adolescents and adults. If periodontal disease is observed, the dentist should decide what radiographs need to be taken, but typically they include selected bitewing or periapical views. Generally toothless adults do not need to have radiographs done.

Situations where radiographs might be taken

Occasionally dental radiographs are taken simply to monitor the growth and development of the oral and maxillofacial region of a child or adolescent. Clinical judgment is necessary in these instances since repeated radiation exposure is involved. Periapical or panoramic films are often taken in adolescents to gauge the development of the third molars. Radiographs can also be done to look at dental implants (or potential sites), assess pathological changes, measure periodontal treatment progress, diagnose dental pulp diseases, locate areas that need restoration, or find minerals in decayed areas.

Historical findings or clinical signs that suggest the need for radiographic evaluation
If dental history includes any periodontal or endodontic (pulp) treatment, soreness, or evidence of trauma, radiographs may be needed. X-rays are usually taken when there is familial history of dental problems or there is a need to check demineralization. There are numerous clinical signs that can indicate use of radiographs. In addition to evidence of various types of dental disease, unexplained symptoms in the area like bleeding, sensitivity, discoloration, or eruptions warrant radiographs. Sinus problems, neurological abnormalities or asymmetry in the facial region, and temporomandibular joint (TMJ) problems are just a few other clinical symptoms that dictate probable use of diagnostic radiography.

Predisposition to caries development

There are numerous factors that can predispose a patient to caries development. If patient history, clinical evaluation, or other testing indicates the presence of any of these factors, radiographs are probably necessary. Evidence of poor oral hygiene or insufficient fluoride use, excessive drug or alcohol use, or a diet heavy in sugar content all increase the possibility of caries. Previous history of decay, demineralization, dental restorations, dry mouth, and chemo- or radiation therapy all increase the risk of caries development. The mouth can be swabbed and titers of bacteria that commonly cause caries can be taken to assess risk as well. A child that has been nursed excessively is more disposed to caries formation.

Reduce occupational radiation exposure

The dental technician or other personnel operating a dental x-ray machine must stand in a position that shields them from the useful x-ray beam as well as potential radiation leakage from the tubehead or scatter from interaction with the patient. In general, this means that dental professionals need to position themselves at least 6 feet away from the patient and at an angle of between 90 and 135 degrees relative to the x-ray beam. If this is impossible, then the operator must wear a leaded protective barrier or stand behind a wall that is dense and deep enough (such as drywall) to absorb the radiation. Other office personnel should be located outside the wall. Radiation exposure to occupationally as well as non-occupationally exposed employees is usually monitored with a film badge. Individuals wear this film badge, which consists of a lithium fluoride crystal, and periodically a film badge dosimetry monitoring service uses the badge to quantify the person's radiation exposure. The badge should be worn in the neck, chest, or hip area.

Determine whether a protective barrier or wall is adequate radiation protection
A guide number for protective barriers or walls can be calculated as the product of the workload (W) times the use factor (U) times the occupancy factor (T). Workload is expressed in milliampere minutes per week the machine is used, the use factor is determined by the type of surface (wall versus floor or ceiling) and its orientation to the main x-ray beam, and the occupancy factor reflects the percentage of time the individual remains behind the barrier. Thus, the use factor for walls is ¼, much greater than the U for walls or ceilings (1/16). Similarly, the occupancy for regular office personnel right behind the barrier is 1 while the T for individuals in other areas is much less. Concrete, cinder block, and thick drywall are generally acceptable construction materials.

Universal precautions in the dental setting

Universal precautions are a set of safety measures employed in any setting where personnel or patients might be exposed to pathogens that can be transmitted via the blood or saliva. Viruses such as various types of hepatitis (particularly types B and C) and human immunodeficiency virus (HIV) as well as many infectious bacteria are conveyed by blood or saliva. Dental professionals rarely deal with the patient's blood, but they do regularly come into contact with saliva. OSHA has developed the Bloodborne Pathogen (BBP) Rule, and this federal agency can fine medical or dental facilities that do not adhere to the rules. Most states have a State Board of Dental Examiners (BDE) that also enforces guidelines set up by OSHA and other agencies like the American Dental Association (ADA) and the Centers for Disease Control (CDC). The dental healthcare worker must abide by these rules, but responsibility rests with the employer.

Personal protective equipment in dentistry

Personal protective equipment includes impermeable gowns, masks, disposable gloves, and protective eyewear. All of these are usually worn by healthcare workers in many medical settings and in dentistry if the patient is possibly infectious. Examples of the latter include presence of any respiratory infection like a cold or evidence of coughing and possible discharge of fluid aerosols. The one piece of personal protective equipment that is now recommended in all dental settings including radiographic film positioning and any other intraoral contact is a pair of disposable gloves.

Dental processing solutions

The radiographic developer and fixer solution can sustain microbial growth if present for up to 2 weeks. Therefore, intraoral film should be handled aseptically prior to processing to avoid bacterial load. Panoramic films can become contaminated by contact with the biteblock. If the biteblock is wrapped with a plastic barrier, then the wrapping should be properly discarded after use. The biteblock should be placed in a container and decontaminated after each use. Apparatus involved with panoramic and extraoral filming should be periodically disinfected as well.

Surfaces and decontamination

A classification system originally developed by E. H. Spaulding breaks down the level of decontamination required for infected objects. In dental radiology, theoretically none of the apparatus or equipment used falls into the highest critical category. This classification includes contact with blood products or breaching of tissue, and equipment must either be sterilized or disposed of. Most equipment used in oral and maxillofacial radiology falls into the semicritical category because it is in contact with mucous membranes but does not penetrate the tissues. While sterilization procedures are preferred for semicritical items, high-level disinfection measures or barriers can be used. Equipment employed in panoramic or extraoral radiography often falls into the noncritical category because while it may come into contact with intact skin, it generally does not touch mucous membranes or saliva, nor does it breach the surrounding tissue. Noncritical items as well as environmental surfaces that the patient does not touch should be sanitized, disinfected with mid-range level products, or protected by barriers.

Sanitization vs. disinfection

The terms sanitization and disinfection are often used interchangeably. Both terms indicate the use of some type of removal and cleaning procedure to reduce microbial load. Disinfection involves physical or chemical measures to destroy microorganisms. Semicritical items require high-level disinfection, which is defined as the ability to destroy the bacteria causing tuberculosis. In practice, the surfaces of dental equipment should be sanitized and disinfected at the beginning and end of each day (and if contaminated during the day). Types of disinfectants include phenols, sprays containing an alcohol-phenol mixture, chlorine, and iodophors. Barriers that are changed often can be used as well. Sterilization procedures, on the other hand, destroy all microbes, including viruses, bacteria, and fungi. Most sterilization processes involve steam or dry heat at very high temperatures and pressures.

Infection control procedures

There are three acceptable methods of handling film to reduce the possibility of infection. The least desirable procedure is the overglove method, in which a plastic overglove is aseptically put over the contaminated powder-free latex glove only during transport to the darkroom, films are placed into the processor with clean, bare hands, and another pair of gloves is donned before darkroom cleaning is performed. A better procedure is the three-glove method. Here contaminated films are placed in a cup, the initial contaminated gloves are removed in the x-ray apparatus room, films are taken to the darkroom or loader ungloved after washing, another pair of gloves is put on to unwrap the films there, and equipment cleaning procedures are performed using a third set of gloves. There are also films available that come in plastic barrier pouches that shield the actual film from contact with saliva, or these types of envelopes can be purchased. After the radiograph is taken, the pouches are opened into a cup or onto a paper towel, and then they are taken to the darkroom with washed, bare hands.

Three-glove vs. barrier envelope

The x-ray operator needs to disinfect their hands at several stages during the three-glove or barrier envelope methods of exposure. In practice, the operator disinfects their hands by soap washing; simple hand soaps can be used but soaps containing 4% chlorhexidine gluconate or 3% parachlorometaxylenol are

recommended. Before the procedure, it is preferable to have the patient take off dental hardware and eyewear and rinse their oral cavity with an antimicrobial rinse including chlorhexidine gluconate, some type of phenol, or the herb sanguinarine. The technician dons the initial pair of gloves, and then they briefly examine the patient's oral cavity, set machine parameters, open the sterile film holder and attach the film, and set up the positioning device. Parts of the machine that are touched should be covered with plastic. The exposure should be activated with a foot switch or a plastic-covered button. Films are dropped into separate paper cups (after barrier removal if present), the initial glove is removed, and the technician washes their hands and transports the cup to the darkroom or loader.

Radiographic film packet and removal

Plastic film envelopes if present are removed and wiped of saliva (preferably with disinfectant) before transportation to the darkroom and are not part of the actual film packet. Typical radiographic film packets all have four components. The radiographic film is surrounded by black light-proof paper and backed by a sheet of lead foil. The whole package is enclosed with a moisture and light-proof barrier packet which has a color coded end. In the darkroom, the film is removed by holding that part of the packet and pulling back the black tab to remove the film with its black-paper covering. The film is shaken out of the black paper over a paper towel before development.

Darkroom infection control

Using the preferred three-glove method in the darkroom, exposed films are dropped from the paper cups used for transportation onto a paper towel. The technician then puts a new pair of powder-free gloves over clean hands and removes the film. The film itself is never touched, and it is dropped onto a second paper towel. The technician discards the gloves, rewashes their hands, and processes the film with bare hands being careful to touch only the edges. Handwashing after the processing is also recommended. If a daylight loader is used instead of a manual or automatic processor, the main difference is that the operator works through sleeves that go into the daylight loader and films are usually dropped into cups before loading. Disinfecting and infection control procedures and film removal techniques are similar except that wrappings are initially discarded in the chamber instead of the waste bin as in done in the darkroom. A third pair of gloves must be donned during cleanup.

Infection control after x-rays

For dental radiation procedures, all of the contaminated disposables like gloves, paper towels, and film packets are not defined as infectious materials and can therefore be thrown out in the regular waste. Most other exposed equipment does need to be cleaned or in some cases sterilized. In particular, contaminated film holders must initially be put into temporary solutions and later be subjected to other procedures that decontaminate and sterilize them. For sterilization, the holders can be put in bags with other contaminated dental equipment and then the bags are autoclaved (steam sterilized) or put in a dry-heat oven. Plastic wrap covering switches or other parts of the x-ray machine can be replaced or sprayed or swabbed with a disinfectant, and lead aprons and collars should be disinfected as well. A third pair of gloves should be worn during these procedures. Gowns or protective eyewear if worn should be regularly laundered or disinfected respectively.

Antibiotic use and immunization

In dentistry, there is a small risk of exposure to blood products. Any invasive treatment could theoretically cause bleeding in the patient. While dental radiography is usually not invasive, the patient typically undergoes other oral probing by the dentist at the same visit. Therefore, a patient may be pre-

medicated with antibiotics prior to an oral procedure, particularly if they have a history of certain cardiac diseases or artificial joint replacement. Dental personnel should be immunized against tetanus, influenza, varicella, and hepatitis B virus (HBV) because of their potential exposure to infectious blood products.

Infection control and panoramic radiography

Panoramic radiography is not invasive. The technician can perform the technique with clean, ungloved hands and theoretically does not need any personal protective equipment during the procedure. The patient should wear a leaded apron, however. The bite guide should either be disposable or can be covered with a plastic bag. Patient cooperation is required because they should use an antibacterial mouthwash and perform the actual placement and removal of the biteblock or its covering. After the radiography is performed, equipment that was touched by the patient such as rests or guides should be cleaned.

Intraoral radiographs

There are three types of intraoral radiographs, periapical, bitewing, and occlusal. In a periapical radiograph, the goal is to show the location and outlines and distance from the central jaw arch of the teeth into the surrounding tissue area. The entire tooth and root including minimally 2mm of the periapical bone should be recorded. Bitewing radiographs are held in place with tabs or holding apparatuses during exposure, and they are designed to show the scope of the crown or visible part of the tooth covered by enamel as well as a portion of the bone and roots in the jaw. Bitewing x-rays are useful for observation of calcium deposits, configuration of the pulp area, decay, periodontal issues, and the like. Their advantage is proximity to the teeth and the favored perpendicular beam orientation. Combinations of periapical and bitewing radiographs are combined to take a complete-mouth (CMX) or full-mouth (FMX) x-ray survey. There are also occlusal radiographs that look at the cutting edge surfaces of the teeth and the planes in the mouth; these are useful for observation of obvious abnormalities in the oral cavity.

Upper and lower jaw configuration

In the upper jaw or maxilla, most teeth are angled outward from the jaw. This configuration is known a buccal or facial tilt. In the lower jaw or mandible, the angle between the teeth and the jaw typically changes from a buccal tilt in the front six teeth to an almost upright orientation at the premolars to a small inward or lingual tilt at the back. The real axis of the root of a tooth is the line between the tip of the root, which is not visible to the eye, and the end of the visible part of the tooth. Assumptions about the location of the tip or apical area of the root in the maxilla can be made by envisioning a line between the tragus, the bulge anterior to the ear opening, and the ala or wing of the nose and extrapolating to identifying facial features. The line for similar extrapolation to the mandible is about a half centimeter below the jaw.

Patient's head during periapical radiography

Generally a patient is seated erect during periapical radiography. This position places the plane of the teeth parallel to and the sagittal or right/left midline plane of the head perpendicular to the ground. All points along the aga-tragus line (also known as the maxillary orientation line) should be equidistant from the floor plane for maxillary bone radiographs. The patient's head should be inclined slightly backward during the mandibular shots to rectify the angle changes that occur when the mouth is opened. If muscles on the floor of the mouth become taut, the patient should be instructed to swallow to relax them. Chair height adjustments are often necessary to ensure proper positioning and operator comfort.

Source to film distance is long in periapical radiographs

Of the two periapical radiographic techniques, the paralleling technique is generally preferred over the bisecting angle technique because there is less distortion with paralleling. This decrease in distortion is accomplished by holding the film parallel to the long axes of the teeth and directing the beam perpendicular to both. In order to achieve this parallel orientation, the distance between the film and the teeth usually needs to be increased, which could theoretically decrease the image clarity. Therefore, sharpness and magnification are usually restored by increasing the distance between the x-ray beam source and the film. For this reason, longer 16 inch positioning devices are often utilized.

Angulation of the x-ray beam

The tubehead of the x-ray machine is oriented both vertically and horizontally relative to various planes during periapical radiography. The occlusal plane along the top ridge of the teeth should be placed parallel to the floor, and the tube head height is changed to accommodate this. This vertical angulation is calculated in degrees and is either positive if it angles downward or negative if it angles upward. The angle of the beam is also quantified in terms of its angle from the sagittal plane. In other words, beams directed at back teeth have greater horizontal angles than in the front. This horizontal angulation is determined by the location of the targeted teeth. If feasible, the horizontal angle of the beam should also be parallel to the floor and the flat plane of the film. The beam should be aimed at the desired area or point of entry, and it should cover the entire location of the x-ray film.

Film holders

Rectangular collimation is preferable for the paralleling technique because it directs the x-ray beam in a rectangle, which is the same shape of the film. It limits unnecessary radiation exposure but restricting the area of the beam in contact with the patient. Some x-ray machines have built-in rectangular collimators or positioning devices with rectangular outlets. Several commercial film-holders achieve rectangular collimation by attachments that either fit on the end of the beam indicating device or are integral parts of the film. Masel Precision Instruments manufactures holders of the second variety. Dentsply/Rinn makes both types as well as a disposable polystyrene holder that has markings enabling the operator to position it at different places depending on the desired film. The same manufacturer also produces plastic film holders (proprietary name Snap-A-Ray) that are unbacked and fit directly into the mouth; the disadvantages of these holders are possible breakage, image distortion, and difficulty obtaining the correct angles without an alignment device.

Snap-A-Ray film holders

Snap-A-Ray plastic film holders by Dentsply/Rinn are unbacked Thus they provide less irritation and are generally better tolerated. This makes this type of film holder particularly useful in pediatric patients, individuals susceptible to gag reflexes, and situations where distortion is not a great issue. The latter situations include evaluations of toothless individuals or dental pulp (endodontic) disease. Teeth further back in the mouth are often appraised using these types of holders because it is easier to arrange the film parallel to the teeth. Thus, premolars and molars in the lower jaw or mandible as well as third molar projections of either jaw are often looked at using devices like the Snap-A-Ray film holders.

Good film placement

In the paralleling technique, there are six rules for superior technique and the first three involve placement of the film. The first rule is that the film should include all teeth in the area to be covered. Secondly, the juxtaposition of the tooth's long axis and the film's vertical axis should be parallel. Since the apical or top edge of the tooth must be included, this rule dictates that the expected distance between the tooth and film must often be increased. This increased distance should be used for visualization of teeth in the back of the upper jaw. The front incisors in both jaws tend to tilt outwards, and films of these regions need to be positioned relatively far back in the oral cavity. The third tenet is that the horizontal plane of the film should be at the same angle as the mean tangent for the region; the tangent is flat plane connecting the two end points in the small area being x-rayed.

Good positioning of the beam indicating device

First, this device should be angled vertically with its flat open end parallel to the film container in order to avoid distortion. The positioning tube should also be angled horizontally to the plane of the area to be covered, thus aiming the x-rays perpendicular to the film. Lastly, the center of the cone of x-rays must be localized over the middle of the film in order to avoid partial images or an incomplete pattern known as cone-cutting.

X-rays of the anterior regions of the upper jaw

X-rays of the front or anterior regions of the upper maxillary jaw are typically performed using a plastic anterior biteblock that holds the film package attached to a stainless steel rod that lines up the positioning device and the film. In order to avoid cone-cutting, there is usually a ring that can also be attached to the rod to center the BID and the film. A No. 1 film is usually inserted vertically into the bite block with the plain face outwards. The desired exposure parameters are set on the x-ray machine. The film is centered over a particular tooth depending on the region being radiographed, the maxillary midline for central incisors, the lateral incisor for that region, or the canine for that area. The long axis of the targeted tooth should be parallel to the film. A cotton roll is placed between the biteblock and the teeth in the lower jaw. The aiming ring on the indicator rod is slid down to touch the patient's skin, and vertical as well as horizontal angulation is established before the exposure is taken.

X-rays of the pre-molar and molar regions of the upper jaw

For the pre-molar and molar regions of the upper maxillary jaw, the plastic posterior periapical biteblock is generally used with a No. 2 film. In these maxillary areas, the holder is placed horizontally to either center the second premolar (premolar region) or to have the second premolar at the front edge of the film (molar region). Part of the canine should be included for the second premolar shot. Sometimes the molar projection is moved further back to visualize third molars that have not erupted yet. The film should be aligned parallel to the tangent of the region horizontally and to the long axis of the desired teeth vertically. The bite block is held in place by positioning it against the biting surface of the teeth, inserting a cotton roll below it in the mandible, and instructing the patient to bite down to keep it in place. The aiming ring if present is pulled down to touch the patient's skin, and the positioning device is aligned horizontally and vertically before exposure.

Lower jaw vs. the upper jaw

The same plastic biteblocks and film numbers are used for similar regions in the maxillary and mandibular jaws. The position of the film holder needs to be inverted. For the incisors in the mandible, the film packet is placed relatively far back near the premolars in

order to align the long axis of the teeth in parallel to it. The holder is centered in much the same manner as for the equivalent area of the maxilla. In the mandibular molar region, the third molar should be covered and the film should be put in the groove between the teeth and the tongue. The cotton roll is placed between the biteblock and the corresponding maxillary teeth. As in the radiographs for the upper jaw, the aiming ring is placed next to the skin, the positioning device is aligned horizontally and vertically, and the exposure is taken.

Premolar and molar bitewing radiographs

Number 2 films are typically used for bitewing radiographs of the posterior regions of the oral cavity. They are placed horizontally in the bitewing holder. Exposure parameters are selected. The film holder is held in place by placing it on the hard occlusal surfaces of the bottom teeth and biting down. The premolar bitewing radiograph is centered in the areas that would be covered by both upper and lower premolar periapical films. The molar bitewing is held similarly, and is placed far enough back to cover all three molars. The aiming ring is slid into place near the patient's skin, the positioning device is aligned both horizontally and vertically, and the exposure is taken.

Holders designed for bitewing

Instruments designed for bitewing radiographs typically have a tab or wing connected to the rough grainy side of the film packet. This tab is used to bite down on and hold the film in place. The tab is positioned on the hard surface of either the molars or premolars (depending on the desired shot) of the lower jaw with the film between the teeth and tongue. In order to accomplish this, the technician must initially insert the apparatus by keeping part of the tab against the front of the tooth with one index finger while keeping the film portion vertical with the other one. The patient then closes their teeth down on this wing while the operator keeps the tab portion in place. Separate bitewings for the premolar and molar regions using standard size bitewing films (No. 2.2 usually) are generally performed, with the front edges positioned at either the canine or second premolar respectively.

Vertical and horizontal angulation

Most positioning devices for bitewings are round. If the BID device is short with an 8-inch distance between the x-ray source and the film, it is generally aimed at approximately +10 degrees to the tab. This is because the film tends to angle slightly back from the upper teeth that tilt back, and this vertical angulation establishes a perpendicular relationship between the x-ray and film. For a long BID with a source to film distance of around 16 inches, the angle can be reduced to 8 degrees for a molar bitewing and 6 degrees for a pre-molar bitewing. The flat surface of the positioning device should be parallel to the film. As always, the central portion of the x-ray beam should be aimed at the middle of the film packet.

Isometry and the bisecting angle technique

The rule of isometry asserts that two triangles are equivalent when they have a shared side and two equal angles. Extrapolation of the rule of isometry in the bisecting angle technique results in the assumption that the central portion of the x-ray can therefore be aimed perpendicular to the line that bisects the angle between the film and the long axis of the tooth (the shared side of the two triangles). In reality, distortion is still quite likely when applying this rule because teeth are not flat planes. Therefore the bisecting angle must be strictly observed. If the perpendicular orientation of the BID is close to the angle of the tooth, the image will appear elongated. If the perpendicular orientation of the positioning device is close to the film instead, a phenomenon called foreshortening can occur.

Good bisecting angle technique

First, the head must be correctly positioned for a bisecting angle radiograph. For shots of the maxillary teeth, the plane of the teeth being documented should be parallel and the dividing plane of the head should be perpendicular to the floor. Radiographs of the mandible are taken with the mouth open necessitating inclination of the head backward to keep the plane of the head parallel to the floor. The centers of the film and area to be documented should be superimposed. The middle of the x-ray beam should be angled vertically in the center of the field perpendicular to the bisecting line. The horizontal angulation is determined by directing the beam at right angles to the tangent in the area being documented. The point of entry should be the middle of the desired area.

Vertical angulations of the positioning device

The vertical angulation is the angle between the positioning or beam indicating device and the occlusal plane of the teeth. For the bisecting technique, this angle is always positive for examination of maxillary teeth and usually negative for shots of mandibular teeth. The appropriate angle for short 8-inch positioning devices can vary but starting points ranging from $+30^0$ for molars up to $+55^0$ for incisors are generally used. The angles are slightly less for longer 16-inch BIDs. When documenting mandibular teeth with this method, the vertical angulation usually ranges from 0^0 for molars to about -20^0 for incisors for the short BID and slightly less for the longer devices. Dentsply/Rinn manufactures anterior and posterior holders called BAI for the bisecting angle technique that facilitate the determination of angulation and their Stabe holders can be used for this technique as well.

Oral cavity that affect radiography

A number of anatomical variations or sensitivities that may be present in the oral cavity can affect the use of radiography. Film positioning is difficult for shots of the lower jaw in individuals with large tongues, for example. If the roof of the mouth is shallow, it may be difficult to maintain a parallel relationship between the film and the long axes of the teeth in the upper jaw; vertical angulation may need to be increased and the probability of a foreshortened image will be increased. There are several types of common bony outgrowths or exostoses that can create problems. About one-fifth of the population has this type of growth in the middle of their hard palate (torus palatinus) and a smaller proportion of people have similar growths on the lower jaw (torus mandibularis). In both cases, the film should not be placed over the bony growth. Some people have very sensitive mucous membranes or high muscle attachments in the area around the premolars of the lower jaw, and film placement may need to be adjusted accordingly. Sensitivity in the mandibular incisor area is also common. Lastly, some patients will be fully or partially edentulous, and exposure times for these individuals can be minimal.

Alleviating pain and anxiety

Some patients are anxious or tend to experience discomfort during radiography. If all desired areas can be visualized on a panoramic radiograph, its substitution for intraoral procedures can alleviate anxiety and discomfort. Sometimes films used for intraoral radiography can be bent if the inflection does not mask the teeth being documented. There are ways to relax the muscles in the area being x-rayed. These include placing the film closer to the tongue or using commercially available tissue pads attached to the top edge of the film. Anesthetics can be applied topically to the region, but they should be rinsed out after the dental procedures. Occasionally, patients are given prescription tranquilizers like diazepam to reduce their apprehension.

Gag reflex

The gag reflex is a natural defense mechanism in which a person coughs and vomits in an attempt eject foreign objects and keep airways open. The reflex is activated by touching an object in the oral cavity such as the x-ray film, but it can also be produced by mental or emotional fears about the process. Confidence on the part of the operator is a big help in suppressing the gag reflex. Speed, placement, and the order of placement are all important as well. This is particularly true for placement of the film in the maxillary molar region because gagging is most likely to occur at that time. Use of biteblocks or other holding apparatuses can sometimes dispel the reflex. Techniques such as deep nose breathing or hypnosis may alleviate the gag reflex. Topical anesthetics are used occasionally as well.

What occurs during gag reflex
The gag reflex is the tendency to choke or vomit. A portion of dental patients will experience this tendency during dental procedures such as radiography. The reflex is initiated when its receptors, which are located on the back third of the tongue as well as the rear of the throat, are irritated. Nerves located in these regions send messages to the gag center in the medulla oblongata portion of the brain. Nerves from the brain transmit signals to muscle fibers associated with the gag reflex. Initially, the patient cannot breath, and later muscles in the upper part of the abdominal cavity and the upper portion of the throat contract. This choking reaction may be accompanied by regurgitation of undigested food as well.

Reducing the gag reflex in a patient
The tendency of a patient to experience a gag reflex can be reduced by elimination of stimuli that either increase anxiety or create irritation of the oral cavity. The demeanor of the dentist or x-ray technician can greatly influence the anxiety level of the patient. The specialist can reduce psychic or perceived stimuli by maintenance of professional

behavior, use of ways to divert attention like talking, involvement of the patient in performance of the task, or x-ray documentation of the most sensitive areas last. The patient can also be given tranquilizers to reduce the reflex. Hypersensitivity or tactile stimuli can be reduced by careful placement of the holder and rapid exposure of the film. Measures to reduce the hypersensitivity may be required such as locally applied anesthetics or cold water or placement of salt on the end of the tongue.

Maxillary topographic projection

A maxillary topographic projection is a type of occlusal radiograph designed to document a large portion of the upper jaw. Higher speed, large occlusal film packets and longer 16-inch positioning devices are generally utilized. The smaller potential difference of 65 kVp and 15 mA current are the usual exposure factors. The film is positioned far back in the mouth with the rough surface against the maxillary teeth, and the patient holds it in place by biting down. The aga-tragus line should be parallel to and the midsagittal plane should be at right angles to the ground. The theory of bisecting angles is used to take the x-ray, which means that the central portion of the x-ray beam is directed perpendicular to the bisecting line between the planes of the film and the upper incisors. In order to achieve this angulation, the positioning device is usually placed about +65 degrees to the film plane near to but not touching the nose.

Mandibular symphysis projection

A mandibular symphysis projection is a type of occlusal radiograph designed to document a large area of the incisor region of the lower jaw. The film is placed with the rough side facing the occlusal surfaces of the mandible. In this procedure, the patient's head is inclined backward to form a 45 degree angle between the floor and the biting surface plane. The midline plane should be perpendicular to the ground. The bisecting angle technique is employed to center the x-ray beam. This translates to an angle between the film and x-ray of about 55° and a vertical angulation of about -20 degrees. The beam indicating device is usually placed against the chin.

Mandibular cross-sectional projection

A mandibular cross-sectional projection is a type of occlusal radiograph used to document the presence of bodies like stones or calcified areas in glands in the lower jaw area. Settings are similar to those used for mandibular symphysis projections, but the head is tilted much further back until the plane of the maxillary teeth is actually upright and perpendicular to the floor. The film is positioned with the rough surface against the mandibular teeth and centered along the midline. Its back edge should be placed against the front of the rami or branching parts of the cavity. The middle part of the x-ray beam is directed at right angles to the occlusal film by positioning the BID close to but not touching the lower chin.

Posterior occlusal projections

Posterior occlusal topographic projections can be taken for both the upper and lower jaws. For the maxillary jaw, this type of film is useful for visualization of the sinus and other structural areas in the posterior or back. In this case, the film is placed lengthwise along the midline on one side of the face, the patient bites down on it, and the positioning device directs the x-ray beam at about a 55 degree angle through the profile near the premolar region. For the mandible, separate projections for each side of the mouth are usually unnecessary, but if they are required the film can again be placed on one side with the long edge positioned anteroposteriorly along the center. Here the film packet should touch the ramus of the lower jaw, and the beam still needs to be directed perpendicular to the film.

Temperature control in manual processing of radiographs

The effective temperature range for the manual processing of x-rays is between 60°F and 75°F, and the suggested temperature is 70°F. Above this temperature range fogging can occur due to excessively rapid development, and below this range both development and fixation proceed too slowly. At 70°F, film density and contrast are fairly ideal and the processing time is convenient. This temperature can be sustained easily in the master water bath or rinsing tank by a mixing valve that combines the hot and cold water coming in. Typically, 2 different insert tanks for either developing or fixing chemicals are put into this tank. A thermometer should be clipped to the tank to ensure maintenance of the proper temperature, and a timer should be used to control development and fixation intervals.

Safelight and parameters

A safelight is a weak light used with filters in a darkroom to enable the technician to process radiographs without excessive fogging. The wattage of the bulb is very low, typically between 7.5 and 15 watts if it directly illuminates the area and up to 25 watts if the lighting is indirect. The light source should be at least 4 feet from the processing area, and processing time should be kept to 8 minutes or less. Filters are placed between the light source and the processing area to screen out portions of the light spectrum. Amber or red filters are most often utilized because the yellow and red region is complementary to the most sensitive colors for x-ray film, blue and green light. Currently, the most commonly used filter is the red Kodak GBX-2, which is suggested for higher E and F speed films of the oral cavity as well as extraoral films that contain rare-earth substances that emit light when irradiated.

Manual processing of x-rays

Lock the darkroom. Label processing hangers. Agitate developer and fixing solutions with individual stirrers and chemicals; refill if necessary. Check temperature of the water bath; adjust if necessary by means that will not dilute the solution. All white light should be eliminated; activate safelight. Using gloves, open the film packet. Remove gloves; insert films into their hangers. Adjust interval timer to the development time (usually 5 minutes for a 70°F bath). Lower film into the developer solution; begin timing. Initially, rapid agitation up and down is suggested to get rid of air bubbles and saturate the film surfaces. At the end of the development period, the film is transferred to the rinsing tank (water bath) and swirled for about a half minute to remove developer. The film is put into the fixer solution for approximately twice the development time, typically 10 minutes. After fixation, normal lighting can be turned on and the safelight turned off. The film is washed in the bath for 15 to 20 minutes, dried on a rack, and then mounted.

Typical manual developer solution

The primary purpose of the developer solution is to reduce the silver halide crystals generated during the radiation into black metallic silver. Usually, the reducing agents employed are metol, which acts rapidly to induce gray tones, and hydroquinone, which acts more gradually but generates better contrast. Developer solutions also contain an activator like sodium carbonate, which provides an alkaline pH and also softens the emulsion. The solutions include an agent called a restrainer that prevents the non-exposed silver bromide crystals from developing and producing unwanted fog; typically potassium bromide is used. Lastly, developers contain a preservative such as sodium sulfite; the role of the preservative here is to stop the solution from oxidizing. All of the chemicals are dissolved in water.

Typical manual fixer solution

The purpose of fixation is to remove unexposed silver halide crystals and terminate the development process. The fixing or clearing agents that remove the unexposed silver bromide crystals from the emulsion gel are typically thiosulfates coupled to either ammonium or sodium. The acidic medium that actually terminates the development by neutralization is usually either acetic or sulfuric acid. A preservative like sodium sulfite is included as well to prevent the breakdown of the fixing agent. In addition, a chemical that shrinks and hardens the gelatin is added; examples of hardeners are aluminum chloride, aluminum sulfide, and potassium aluminum sulfate. All of the chemicals are dissolved in water.

Wet reading

In emergencies, a manually processed radiograph can be wet read. This means that the radiograph is removed from the fixer early and observed near the safelight. Actual clearing of the solution means that the cloudy appearance of the film had disappeared and the silver halide crystals have been converted. This reaction takes about 2 minutes which means that a wet reading can be taken shortly thereafter (3 or 4 minutes of fixation) if necessary. For permanent documentation, however, recommended fixation times should be employed. A short fixation time (such as termination after wet reading) means that the emulsion is not hardened enough, drying will be prolonged, and the image may be lost with aging. Alternatively, too long a fixation time can result in irreversible binding of the fixer to the gel and subsequent brown discoloration of the radiograph.

Manual vs. automatic processing

When an automatic processor is used, the total processing time is greatly reduced over manual methods. The total time involved can be as little as one and half to 5 minutes. This time reduction is achieved through use of rollers that guide the film through the processor and wring out excess solutions as well as by increasing the temperature and the concentrations of reagents. Some chemical substitutions and additions are made as well. The reducing agent in the developer is changed to phenidone instead of metol because the former works faster in conjunction with the hydroquinone. Glutaraldehyde is typically added to the developer to harden the gel, and sulphates are included as well to prevent swelling. The goal is the prevention of sticking to the rollers in the machine. Instead of approximately 70^0F, processing temperature is around 83^0F. Solutions are replenished often by injection into the floor of the tank. Drying is performed in the machine with streams of heated air, and the finished radiograph is automatically dropped onto a platform.

Films in an automatic processor

If the automatic processor has a daylight loader, film packets are opened and fed into the machine inside this loader. Therefore, provisions for keeping light out are unnecessary. If the machine does not have a loader, packets are opened with gloves in a locked darkroom with a safelight. In either case, films are inserted into the processor with bare hands in a very controlled, deliberate manner in order to avoid jamming of the machine. This is particularly essential for panoramic films which are fed lengthwise. For a bent film, the straight side should be introduced first. The time interval between insertions of different films should be at least 5 seconds. Films must be dry when inserted to avoid roller contamination and lines on later films.

Maintenance of automatic processors

Some procedures should be performed daily in order to properly maintain automatic processors. These include replenishment of the solutions as needed depending on the daily development load, maintenance of the suggested temperature, and evaluation of the transport rollers for proper alignment. About twice as much developer relative to fixer is used and needs to be replenished; some machines have infrared sensors that automatically determine the needed replenisher. The automatic processing solutions should be completely changed at intervals appropriate to the workload, which can be as often as weekly in a busy office. When the machine is not being used, the lid should be left slightly ajar to permit fumes to escape and reduce subsequent film fogging. The processor should be cleaned about once a week, and lubricant should be applied to gears, bearings and the like about once a month.

Safe disposal of radiographic waste

When an x-ray is taken and developed, several types of waste are created. The first is solid waste including the radiograph itself. Though the discarding of radiographs is not regulated by the government, silver can be extracted from them by heating them above the melting point of silver. The lead foil inserts from the film package should be returned to the manufacturer for proper disposal. Another type of waste is the discarded fixer solution, which contains silver as well, and whose disposal may be regulated locally. The silver in these solutions can be precipitated out by chemical means or electrolysis. In addition, any waste that may have been contaminated by blood or saliva is considered medical waste and should be sent in marked containers to proper disposal facilities.

Mounting radiographs

The recommended procedure for mounting radiographs is to place them in a relationship as though the viewer is looking straight at the patient. This orientation requires that mounting be done with all the raised dots of the film facing the observer and is sometimes termed labial mounting. Sometimes older readings were done in the opposite orientation (lingual mounting), but that procedure is no longer suggested. A viewbox is used for observation. Radiographs are arranged on it with all raised dots upward and segregated according to anatomical location. They are touched only on the periphery with either clean, dry hands or cotton gloves. Identification of anatomical sites can be aided by the knowledge of various landmarks.

Mounting a full mouth survey

Typically, the back teeth of the upper jaw are arranged first with their crowns facing toward the bottom of the viewbox using landmarks of the dental arch to distinguish pre-molars from molars. Then maxillary teeth toward the front are arranged with their edges facing downward. The incisors are placed in the center with laterals and canines to the appropriate side as identified by landmarks. Similarly, mandibular radiographs are arranged with the crowns or incisal surfaces facing upwards. Bitewing radiographs are then mounted in the middle on the sides with the planes between the two biting edges oriented upward toward the back of the cavity. A useful landmark for these radiographs is the root pattern as molars in the lower jaw have two roots while those in the upper jaw have three.

Duplicating films vs. usual x-ray films

Duplicating films are used to copy previously taken radiographs. These films have undergone a process called solarization which overexposes the film to the point where maximum density is reversed. This is achieved through chemical treatment of the film or bombardment with light. One side of the duplicating film consists of the solarized emulsion on polyester base; it is identified by its purple color. The other side is protected with a layer of dye that absorbs reflected light (halation) to eliminate unsharpness in the copied image; this antihalation layer is typically glossy in appearance. Because the film is a type of direct-reversal film, exposure times affect the density in reverse order to a normal film.

Duplicating radiographs

Radiographs can be copied in the darkroom with safelight illumination. Duplicator machines are commercially available. An ultraviolet light source is directed through the original radiograph onto the purple solarized emulsion surface of the duplicating film. The original and duplicating films must be in intimate contact to avoid blurring of the duplicated image. The initial radiograph is put on the surface of the duplicator or illuminator, and the solarized side of the duplicating film is placed directly on top of it. The cover is closed and the filmed is exposed for the time interval suggested by the manufacturer. After exposure, the film needs to be developed as usual.

Judging image quality

Radiographic image quality is judged by a number of interrelated characteristics. The radiograph should have enough detail to differentiate between various components on the film as well as sufficient definition to show structural characteristics and clear demarcation between the components. In general, the latter characteristic, definition, is adequate when surrounding spaces are distinct from the teeth being documented. While detail is primarily controlled by the potential difference applied and to an extent the development procedures, definition is more a function of factors that can be controlled by the operator such as film speed, movement, or length of the positioning device. The darkness of the film in general is the density, which should be in a range where surrounding tissues can be faintly observed; it is affected by a number of parameters. A related characteristic is contrast, which is the differentiation in densities between adjoining areas, and this factor is primarily determined by the voltage applied. Suitable contrast is important for observation of smaller details and tooth decay. In addition, there should be no significant handling or development errors visible.

Judging in terms of structures documented and absence of distortion

In a full mouth survey, the tip of every tooth and its adjoining bone should be observed on at least one of the x-rays. For documentation of particular regions, all spaces between, surrounding and/or retromolar to the teeth desired should be visible on the film. Partial images as a result of cone cutting are unacceptable. The cutting edge of the tooth should be oriented toward the raised bump on the film. Distortion of the comparative size and shape of structures should be kept to a minimum. For bitewing radiographs, interproximal connections should be distinct, the visible parts of the teeth in both jaws should be in the center, the peak of the alveolar bone should be visible and differentiated from the teeth, and the biting surface of the teeth should be horizontal. On the other hand, the molar ridges or cusps should be somewhat overlapping.

Poor patient preparation and radiographic errors

Patient preparation errors with regard to unacceptable radiographic images generally fall into two categories. The first category is the additional overlapping of radiopaque artifacts. These artifacts result from failure to remove primarily metallic hardware from the body or oral cavity. Examples include dental hardware, many types of jewelry, glasses, and artificial hairpieces. Any type of movement from the patient including touching the equipment can result in unsharpness or blurring of the image by increasing the peripheral penumbra area of the focal spot. Good chairside technique from the technician should eliminate these errors.

Mistakes in film placement and radiographic errors

A common film placement error is the positioning of the packet too shallow to record the entire tooth while leaving quite a bit of blank area near the crown visible. This error usually occurs because the patient experiences discomfort and does not bite down enough. Sometimes the entire region desired is not documented, which is a situation that should not occur if landmark guidelines are followed. If the film has been positioned backwards with the lead foil surface exposed to the x-ray beam, an image will be recorded but there will be a tracking pattern from the foil superimposed on the radiograph and its orientation will be inverted. If the radiolucent raised dot on the film packet is inadvertently placed toward the apices of the teeth, it may be superimposed on the radiograph. Double images will be recorded if a film packet is used twice by mistake. If the tongue or a finger is in the path of the x-ray beam, it will appear as an artifact on the radiograph. All of these errors warrant repetition of the procedure.

Overlapping mistakes

Overlapping on radiographic images can occur as a result of two types of errors. The first type can occur when the flat surface of the film packet is not placed parallel to the mean tangent of the area being documented. As a result, the contacts and openings between the teeth appear to slide over one another or overlap. Incorrect horizontal angulation of the positioning device also can be visualized on a radiograph as overlapping. The most common horizontal angulation error is direction of the beam obliquely, not perpendicularly, to the plane of the film. As a result, definition and density are both diminished. Both types of overlapping errors can be corrected by observing the principle of directing the x-ray cone perpendicular to the mean tangent of the area and keeping the film in the same orientation as the tangent.

Distortion errors

Distortion of shapes on radiographs results from either improper vertical angulation or incorrect placement of the film. Elongation or apparent extension of the tooth image occurs when the vertical angulation used is too small, and the less frequent phenomenon of foreshadowing or apparent reduction of tooth size can happen if the vertical angle used is too large. Distortion sometimes occurs if the film package protrudes in the center due to either excessive biting down by the patient or full or partial removal of the film backing. The relative dimensions of parts of an image can also be distorted when the bisecting angle method is utilized, especially when this technique is applied to documentation of maxillary molars. In this case, the roots are not in the bisecting angle plane and therefore the paralleling method is preferable here.

Blank radiograph and low or high density

If a radiograph is blank, no radiation was delivered. Most often this is due to failure to turn on the machine, use the correct tube head, or activate the exposure button. This situation can also occur if the positioning device was severely malpositioned or the film indicated was not used. If the film has been overfixed or inadvertently left in the water bath for a day or two, it may also be blank or clear because emulsion has been washed off. If the film has clearly been exposed, but is very light, the amount of radiation delivered was insufficient or the film was not completely developed. A number of factors can influence the quantity of radiation given, but underdevelopment is usually due to depletion of developer in the processor. If the developer evaporates and is low in the tank, a partial image may be seen only where the development occurred. High-density, very dark films are generally a result of overexposure.

Artifacts or unwanted deposits

If the exterior of the film is contaminated before development is performed, black artifacts can be found on the final x-ray. Sources of contamination include developer chemicals and other liquids including saliva, stannous fluoride, seepage of light into the film package, or later adherence of films together during fixation. Many black artifacts are due to fingers with developer on them. Artifacts that appear white on the image are also the result of contamination, in this case generally drops of clearing solution, air bubbles, or fingers dipped in fixer solution. A variety of apparent timesavers as well as dirty rollers in the automatic machines can result in black streaks on the radiograph. Chemicals from the processing solutions or present on film hangers can precipitate out of solution and appear as deposits on the radiograph. Depleted reagents during processing or inadequate rinsing can result in staining of the finished radiograph. This phenomenon most commonly occurs when the fixer is not sufficiently removed during the final wash. Here a brown stain occurs over time because silver sulfide is formed from the reaction between hyposulfite and metallic silver. Shrinking or reticulation of the film is possible if it has been exposed to rapid temperature changes.

Artifacts or problems

When a film is inserted into an automatic processor, the machine can jam and stop transporting the film along the processor. There are many reasons for this occurrence, ranging from inadequately hardened gelatin to dirty components to improper feeding. If films are fed into the machine too rapidly, they can stick together producing dark dense spots in those areas. Marks can appear on the surface of the radiograph if the rollers are encrusted or have irregularities or if the film has been improperly handled prior to insertion. Rinse water that is dirty or too low or contaminated clearing solution can generate films that appear chalky. Films should be dry when they exit from the automatic processor, but if they are wet or sticky a number of parameters related to the dryer and temperature controls should be checked. Brown discoloration observed with manual processing can occur with automatic machines, but films can also come out greenish yellow in color if inadequate fixation occurred or processing was too rapid.

Errors during film handling

Pressure marks can be found on incorrectly handled films; these marks can be either black teeth marks or white marks formed by writing on the front of the film packet. Black lines appearing on radiographs are the result of intentional bending of the film to alleviate patient anxiety. If saliva is not removed from the film packet, the black protective paper on the film can stick to the emulsion producing black marks on the radiograph. Black streaks or marks can also be generated on films if static electricity contacts the film; therefore, humidity levels need to be maintained in the darkroom especially during the winter. Lackadaisical handling of films can result in tearing, scratching, or artifacts resulting from contact with powder or other contaminants. The biggest problem that occurs, however, is the undesired density of film fogging. Film fog can result from many types of errors, including light leakage, incorrect use of safelights, unsuitable storage conditions, overdevelopment, and film deterioration.

Quality assurance components

Quality assurance is the summation of administrative and technical steps required to maintain reliable and reproducible results in any type of work setting. In the context of a dental radiological setup, quality assurance efforts translate to practices that will assure consistent, comprehensible radiographs with minimal radiation exposure. There are usually two components to quality assurance. The first component is quality administration, which is the administrative aspect of coordinating efforts to ensure high-quality work. The other part to quality assurance is quality control, which encompasses the actual test procedures and technical practices required to maintain consistent, first-rate results.

Dental facilities are staged

A dental facility is staged according to the type of radiographic equipment, extent of radiography performed, the processing method utilized, and the average weekly volume of films. For example, facilities that do only intraoral radiography receive fewer points than those that do other types as well. Similarly, automatic processing is assigned more points than manual procedures only. Large workloads are allocated higher levels as well. The total of points is added up and the dental practice is considered to be Stage 1 (less than 8 points), Stage II (8 to 11 points), or Stage III (at least 12 points).

The AAOMR recommendations

The AAOMR is the American Academy of Oral and Maxillofacial Radiology, and this organization has established guidelines for quality assurance programs in dental practices based on the staging. Those practices falling into the Stage 1 category have relatively low workload, limited range of types of radiology performed, and probably manual processors. The guidelines recommend that these types of facilities include reference films and a retake log book in their program, along with visual assessment of films every day, inspection of the viewboxes and darkroom every month, and quality control checks for the x-ray apparatus once a year. Stage II practices, with some combination of higher workload, varied types of films and/or an automatic processor, should add checking of the processing solutions every day and evaluation of the cassettes and intensifying screens once a month. AAOMR suggests that Stage III offices, with high workloads and various types of radiography, should also have two types of monitoring equipment available, a sensitometer and a densitometer.

Pocket dosimeter

A pocket dosimeter is a small rod-shaped ionization chamber used to quantify the radiation being emitted from the x-ray machine. It basically consists of an air-filled chamber, a quartz fiber, a lens, and a switch that is charged prior to use. The dosimeter is used to compare radiation produced through a series of exposure settings relative to the same settings at baseline. The number of milliroentgens generated or the relative gray scale on a wedge should be equivalent to the baseline values. If the current readings do not match the reference value, then the timer and the mA circuit must be checked as well. There are commercially available meters to check timers, but this can also be done manually by directing the central x-ray beam perpendicularly to a spinning top apparatus attached to a film and counting the number of dots shown on the film. After checking the timer, the filament or mA circuit can be evaluated in one of two ways. If more than one current setting is available, output in milliroentgens can be measured at the same theoretical mAs product for each; if readings do not match, repair is indicated. With only one mA setting available, outside servicing is required. These procedures should be performed yearly.

Quality control procedures

The potential difference or kVp, the precision of its setting, and the size of the focal spot all influence the quality of the x-ray beam emitted from the machine. These parameters should be checked once a year. The test generally used to evaluate the potential difference or penetrating power of the beam is the half-value layer test. Sheets of aluminum of various thicknesses are placed between the positioning device and a pocket dosimeter. With the x-ray equipment at highest voltage or potential difference, the beam is directed through the aluminum and the output in mR is measured by the dosimeter. Half of the maximal output should pass through a particular disc as outlined by federal guidelines; failure to do so indicates needed repair. Accuracy of the voltage setting is typically checked with commercially available meters. These meters quantify the wavelength and frequency of a beam directed at a target; since potential difference determines these two parameters, its accuracy is ascertained.

Focal spot size and evaluation

The focal spot size is the surface area covered by the x-ray beam. Typically, the spot size deteriorates and becomes larger over time due to constant bombardment with electrons. If the spot size is enlarged, the resolution or ability to differentiate adjoining structures in the image is decreased. Spot size is checked with a simple plastic tube, usually 6 inches in length. The tube has a leaded closed end with slots that the BID is placed against, and an open end that is positioned over a large occlusal film. Exposure is performed and then the resolution on the test film is evaluated by counting the number of line pairs per millimeter that can be resolved. Generally, if the resolution is less than or equal to 7 pairs per millimeter, resolution is inadequate. In this case, either a new machine should be bought, or the tubehead can be reconstructed.

Collimator efficacy

Collimator efficacy should be checked every year. A collimator is a device that limits the shape and size of the x-ray beam. Current standards dictate that the beam must be focused or collimated to a maximum of 2 ¾ inches at the end of the positioning device. There are several ways to perform a collimation test. One method is to direct the end of the positioning device onto either a panoramic cartridge or a rare earth fluorescent screen and expose the screen briefly; the technician then either records the area of fluorescence by looking through the leaded window or develops the panoramic packet. The area of exposure should not exceed the BID's diameter. Alternatively, smaller films can be arranged around the tip of the BID with the device covering about half of each packet, each is exposed simultaneously, and after processing the arrangement is reestablished to see whether total exposure area is within the established guidelines. If examination indicates that the radiation beam is not centered, generally the collimator position can be readjusted or a new one purchased.

Detecting and controlling fog

Every month, a fog check for undesired density and its causes should be performed. The fog or excess density is due to exposure of silver halide crystals as a result of white or undesired wavelengths of light. The basic check is done by turning off every source of light in the closed darkroom. After the technician acclimates to the darkness, they observe and subsequently block off any area where white light seeps into the room. The safelight should also be tested because there is a finite amount of time, generally up to 8 minutes, during which even this light can be on during processing. One procedure called the coin test involves processing a series of pre-exposed films at various time intervals by placing a coin on each film after opening the packets and observing how long it takes before the coin is outlined on the film. The maximum time a safelight can be used corresponds to the time when the coin's ridges are visible on the processed film. Safelight timing for cephalometric or panoramic films can be determined by pulling them out of a box at one-inch intervals per minute, and then checking when a line of density begins to emerge on one of the films (in other words, the maximum time for safelight use).

Monitoring processing solutions

The amount and temperature of processing solutions can affect the density of radiographs. Therefore, related quality control procedures should be performed every day. The best way to accomplish these processing solution checks is to keep a cadre of refrigerated reference films that are opened and run through the processing procedure daily. The reference films have gradated levels of exposure produced placing the film under a step-wedge. Aluminum step-wedges are commercially available or a similar device can be made using lead foil strips. After the processor is brought to the correct temperature for its type, a reference film is processed and then compared to a baseline film that was developed when solutions were fresh. The films are viewed on an illuminator and if the daily contrast and density has degraded relative to the baseline film, solutions should be replenished. Developer and sometimes fixer may need to be added every day if processing volumes are large or contamination occurs. Consequently, in larger Stage III facilities, sensitometers and densitometers are utilized together to generate reproducible images and check them for contrast and density respectively.

Monitoring equipment

Stage I and II practices either perform fewer or less varied types of radiographic procedures than Stage III facilities. Instead of performing a daily step-wedge test, the technicians may use a commercially available quality control device. Currently available devices primarily monitor density changes of reference films relative to a baseline film in terms of standardized density monitoring strips. Previously exposed films and strips with numbered densities are provided in the kit. A reference film is initially developed and assigned a density off the standardized strips by reading in the device. When the other films are processed daily, their density is also measured and numbered. Mismatches that are close are usually related to equipment or exposure settings, whereas larger discrepancies of 2 units or more are usually related to the processing solutions or methodology.

Quality control practices

Auxiliary equipment such as leaded aprons and thyroid jackets, panoramic cassettes, and viewboxes need to be checked at regular intervals. Documentation should include a retake log book which includes explanations of errors for reference and a general quality assurance register that records all procedures, outcomes, and remedial actions taken. Settings for exposure parameters and film speed under all possible scenarios should be clearly displayed in the work area. Charts illustrating time versus temperature for processing and darkroom maintenance procedures and schedules should also be posted. All equipment measurements and manuals should be readily available. Film expiration dates should be monitored.

Billing and patient's rights

There is legal precedence of the opinion that x-rays are owned by the dental facility generating them, not the patient. By themselves, x-rays are of little value to the patient who is not adept at interpreting them. Therefore, billing for radiographs should always be bundled with the cost of dental diagnosis and treatment to avoid the issue of ownership of the x-rays. Negligence claims or malpractice suits can occur if x-rays are delivered to the patient or if they are not applied diagnostically. A radiograph can be submitted as factual evidence in certain legal situations and should therefore always be high-quality. On the other hand, while a dentist is not legally compelled to send completed x-rays to other dentists upon request, they may transmit duplicates via certified or registered mail upon written solicitation by the second practice.

Panoramic and Special Imaging Methods

Rotational panoramic radiography

Rotational panoramic radiography exposes the patient to much less radiation than intraoral procedures; for example a panoramic view utilizes only about 1/10 the dose of a typical full-mouth survey. It also covers a larger area of the dental arches and surrounding tissues. The images generated by panoramic radiography are comparatively free of distortion and there is little overlay of different structures. Since the film is not placed in the mouth, the possibility of infection is greatly reduced. Diagnostically, panoramic radiography offers many advantages, including the decrease in the detection window for decay, periodontal disease, and pulp abnormalities.

Rotation of the x-ray

In rotational panoramic radiography, the x-ray beam is rotated in the horizontal plane through a narrow slit around an imperceptible rotational axis in the mouth. The effective focal spot for this plane is essentially the same area targeted on a normal intraoral projection because the moving positions of the ray cross at that position (also identified as the center of rotation). The vertical plane is not influenced by this rotation so its focal spot corresponds to that generated by the x-ray tube. Typically, the vertical plane is angled slightly negative, about -4 to -7 degrees, to direct that aspect through the base of the skull. The film is also rotated in the opposite direction through a horizontal axis in order to equilibrate the horizontal and vertical magnifications. Otherwise, the horizontal aspect would be exaggerated relative to the vertical.

Tomography and panoramic radiography

Tomography is a radiographic procedure that records images in one plane while obscuring or getting rid of images in the other plane. The concept is actually utilized for a number of techniques, including panoramic radiography, computed tomography (CT), and magnetic resonance imaging (MRI). For rotational panoramic radiography, as the x-ray source and film are rotated around the stationary patient, a tomogram or pantomogram is generated. The unblurred plane is called the focal trough or image layer, and only objects in the center of the intersecting projections will be clear. Therefore, patient positioning is crucial in order to target the desired focal trough.

Image layer on panoramic projections

There is a direct relationship between the width of the image layer and the effective projection radius. The latter term refers to the distance between the beam's rotational center and the central plane of the image. The relatively unblurred image layer will be increased as this radius increases. The width of the slit beam affects the size of the image layer inversely, so narrow slits augment the size of the focal trough. The speed at which the film is moving also influences the focal trough by modifying the relationship the rotational center and the focal spot; faster speeds increase the width of the image layer. The x-ray beam is generally moved in a pattern that shifts the effective rotational center along a desired path depending on the area being documented. This requires keeping the central part of the x-ray beam perpendicular to the tangent of the area at each moving point on the curved path.

Distortions found on panoramic radiographs

During panoramic radiography, the x-ray beam is always projected slightly downward with some negative angulation. Therefore, teeth or other entities that are near to the beam relative to the film will appear somewhat wider and those that are comparatively nearer to the film will seem thinner. Therefore, objects toward the back of the oral cavity may appear slightly larger relative to those in the front. Patient positioning can augment these distortions greatly by shifting the focal layer. Only objects in the central plane appear relatively undistorted.

Structures may appear to be flattened out

A panoramic image is generated on a flat plane. The film cassette has a protective lead front with a slit, and as the x-ray tube rotates the film moves across the slit as well. The facial area being documented is curved, but the film is flat. Therefore, the midsagittal plane is in the middle of the image but the teeth and other structures on either side are somewhat flattened and spread-out. Even structures near to this midline can appear flattened if the patient positioning is incorrect; this is an undesirable condition that may disguise other objects as well.

Objects along the midline may appear as double images

When an anatomical structure or other object is located along the midline, a single image is generated if the entity is between the film and the rotational center of the radiation beam. However, there is a central diamond-shaped area emanating from the midline where the beam can pick up structures twice as it rotates. Objects in this area can appear on the radiograph as double images. One representation is the mirror image of the other but both are real. Anatomical structures that often appear as double images include the hard palate and hyoid bone.

Ghost images on panoramic radiographs

Objects that are situated between the center of rotation and the x-ray source can appear as ghost images on panoramic radiographs. These phantom images are not mirror images. Instead they show up on the opposing side of the radiograph, relatively blurry, and positioned higher than their real location. The vertical plane of these ghosts is particularly fuzzy because it is magnified more than the horizontal component. Ghost images can often be observed when the object is located relatively posterior to the mandible, either internally like the horn of the hyoid bone or the back of the hard palate, or externally like earrings or other jewelry. Real single, real double, and ghost images can all appear on the same panoramic x-ray.

Soft tissues and air spaces on panoramic images

It is generally easier to observe soft tissues on panoramic radiographs that with other types of x-rays. This is due to the fact that these types of tissues like cartilage (or fluid) absorb the radiation and thus can appear as light shadows on the x-ray. Nevertheless, poor technique has occurred if structures like the tongue or nose are visible on the image. On the other hand, air spaces do not absorb the radiation and therefore should be black on the radiograph. These characteristic air spaces are known, such as in the nasopharynx, and the presence of other black areas indicates poor methodology as well.

Relative radiolucencies and radiopacities

Any object in the path of the x-ray beam can produce single, double, or ghost images depending on its orientation. These objects include not only anatomical or other entities located on the patient, but also parts of the machinery. All of these images are superimposed on the radiograph, but certain types of tissues and materials block out others to an extent. Radiopaque objects absorb x-rays and radiolucent entities do not in general. Therefore, black air spaces can make it difficult to see hard tissues. Soft and hard tissues are both relatively radiopaque, but hard tissues absorb the radiation to a greater extent and can obscure soft ones. Soft tissues can mask air spaces, and ghost images can be visible over everything else. These concepts can be used to diagnose pathological conditions because changes in an area generally make that region more radiolucent.

Reading panoramic radiographs

Individuals who read panoramic radiographs must be familiar with a variety of common anatomical landmarks in the maxillofacial region and other areas of the face in addition to the teeth. These landmarks include bones, arch structures, ridge formations, palates, typical air spaces, and the like. They must also be aware of what types of structures can obscure others on the image and conditions that affect the relative radiolucency of objects. A much larger area is covered on a panoramic radiograph than any other type of x-ray. The interplay between the teeth and other structures can be visualized to a large extent which means pathological conditions can be more easily diagnosed.

Zones on panoramic radiograph and hallmarks of good images

The largest zone examined on a panoramic radiograph is the central dentition or array of teeth. In a good image, each tooth is distinct, the array spreads upward toward the back resembling a smile, the sizes and relative overlap of teeth on both sides are similar, the tops of teeth are not cut off, and front teeth should be clear. Above this area is the second zone, or the nose and sinus region. Here the lower bones or turbinates of the nasal passage and corresponding air spaces should all appear to be within the nasal cavity, and the hard palate should be observed in this area with the tongue against it. Nasal cartilage should not be visible. Below the central dentition is the mandibular body area. Not much besides the lower border of the mandible should be observed in this third zone. The four corners of the radiograph comprise two different zones. The upper corners, Zone 4, should have centered rounded condyles in the temporomandibular joint area. The lower corners, Zone 6, should primarily be occupied by the hyoid bone. The areas on the sides of the center are Zone 5, should show each ramus or branching part of the lower jaw and possibly some of the spine.

Operation of a panoramic radiographic machine

While there may be some variations with different machines, in general there are five steps involved in patient positioning and subsequent exposure with panoramic radiography. Generally, the first step is to have the patient bite into the groove of the bite block. If the individual is edentulous, a chin rest can be used instead. This step basically centers the patient and their front teeth. Then guides located on the side of the apparatus are locked in place to steady the patient's head and centralize their rear teeth. The chin is then lowered onto the chin rest, which usually has a slight negative incline equivalent to the upward tilt of the x-ray beam. The cervical spine in the neck is then aligned either by having the individual stand erectly or using any means including pillows to achieve straightening in a sit-down type of machine. The patient is then directed to close their lips and place their tongue against the hard palate and remain still while the technician takes the exposure, which typically lasts up to 22 seconds.

Positioning lights

Most panoramic radiographic machines have several positioning lights that are activated before an exposure is taken to ensure correct placement of the patient. Usually there are two vertical lights, one that should be positioned at the corner of the mouth, and another that is focused along the midsagittal plane which should be perpendicular to the floor. There is also a horizontal light that is usually centered along the Frankfort plane, which is the imaginary projection between the floor of the eye socket or orbit and the ear's auditory meatus. In theory, this line should be parallel to the ground. Some panoramic machines have positioning lights that are supposed to run along the ala-tragus instead.

Errors that occur from incorrect positioning when biting into the groove

If the patient bites too far forward into or up against the front of the bite block, the width of the entire image is shrunk. Thus, the most common potential errors are narrowing or missing the crowns of the front teeth or the visible overlap of the cervical spine in the ramus or condyle areas. Sometimes this forward positioning is done intentionally to diagnose sinus disorders because it also shows the structures in the nasal cavity better. If the patient bites too far back into the groove, the image is widened which means that all the zones other than the bottom corners are significantly affected. Undesirable visualization of soft tissues can occur, the front teeth are widened, the condyles may be eliminated from view, and ghost images may appear in several areas.

Errors that occur if the patient's head is tilted in the machine

The purpose of closing the side guides on a panoramic machine is to ensure that the individual's head will be upright and not tilted. However, if the patient's head is inclined to the side, this will be very obvious on the radiograph. The back teeth are generally wider and the rows further apart on one side. The mandible looks larger on that side as well and its lower edge tilts upwards. The condyle on the same aspect also appears to be bigger and higher than the one on the other side. In addition, it is difficult to discern bony details in the upper zones of the image because they tend to be either shadowy or streaked.

Errors that occur when the chin is angled incorrectly

When the chin is angled downward too much or tipped up too high, the relative curving smile-like configuration of the dentition is changed. An excessive downward chin tilt exaggerates this configuration, while tilting the chin upwards too much destroys this relationship and flattens out the dentition on the image. Consequently the front teeth of the upper jaw are either quite prominent or their tops are not seen. Front teeth in the lower jaw either have their apices obscured or they are very clear. Sometimes these errors are deliberately exploited to improve the image quality in those areas. In addition, when the chin is tipped too low, the mandible tends to be drawn out vertically in the front and shows images of the hyoid bone and the condyles may be cut off. If the chin is angled too high, the nasal-sinus cavity can be seen as a large primarily radiopaque area and the condyles may again be eliminated from the image.

Errors that occur when the patient is not correctly positioned upright

The cervical spine in the patient's neck should be straightened before exposing a panoramic radiograph. Sometimes the patient's chin ends up not being against the chin rest. This does not affect the documentation on the central dentition area of the radiograph, but structures normally on the top third of the x-ray are cut off and little is seen on the bottom third. If the individual is slumped over and the spine is not straight, a ghost image of the spine tends to obscure other structures, primarily the front teeth in the central dentition zone as well as parts of the lower jaw.

Errors that occur during the exposure step

During the exposure step, there are basically three kinds of errors that might occur. If the patient does not close their lips and place their tongue against the palate as directed, air between the lips masks the crowns of the front teeth and another air space in the palatoglossal region between the tongue and palates obscures the apices and bone in the maxillary jaw. If the patient moves during the exposure, the main radiographic errors

- 134 -

observed are waves or other distortions in the mandible. Mistakes in the actual exposure process can be made also; typical examples include double exposure, density errors due to incorrect potential difference applied, and labeling mistakes.

Lead apron for panoramic exposure

In panoramic radiography, a leaded apron that looks like a poncho covering both the front and the back is used. This is required to block rays to both the front and back during the rotational pattern of the x-ray beam. However, unlike most other types of exposure, a thyroid collar should not be worn and the apron should not extend into the thyroid area. The beam in panoramic procedure is angled slightly upward and would be projected into shields in the thyroid region resulting in clear, non-exposed parts on the radiograph. Radiation exposure is not a significant problem, however, since total dosage used in the panoramic technique is considerably less than with a complete intraoral series.

Removing most intraoral and extraoral items

If they are not removed, most intra- and extraoral items in the facial regions will show up on the panoramic image as both real and ghost images. The only type of intraoral item that might be left in is acrylic dentures in the front part of the mouth in order to maintain proper interrelationships in that area and steady the patient. Any extra oral item has the potential to disrupt the image, and most should also be taken off. Artificial hairpieces, hearing aids, or eye prosthesis are occasionally left in place.

Procedural errors that affect the quality of panoramic radiographs

One common procedural error is beginning at the wrong place during exposure. This results in loss of part of the anatomic region desired, which shows up on the radiograph as a blank area. Another procedural mistake is failure to remove thick clothing, to place the lead apron correctly, or to adjust for individuals with short necks or broad shoulders. In this case, as the cassette rotates around it may find resistance when it touches the individual. When this disengagement occurs, a vertical band of the film will be overexposed and dark. Some dental offices take out the bite block or other parts (a practice that is discouraged), which can cause a number of radiographic errors including lack of clear separation between rows of teeth and malpositioning of the patient.

Damaged films, screens, and cassettes

Panoramic film will crimp if it has been removed in a rough manner from either the box or the cassette. In this case, a small area of the emulsion is destroyed which shows up on the radiograph as a black, curved mark. Certain types of softer, more flexible cassettes have screens that are pulled out and folded back for film placement. Here, the potential for damage and eventual fissures in the screen is great. Scratches or foreign objects like lint or paper can occur on screens that have not been inspected as well. White lines or spots will appear on the x-ray in all of these types of screen damage because fluorescence during exposure will be prevented in these areas. Cassette damage generally results in light leaks that show up on the film as overexposed, black regions. The more bendable types of cassettes made of vinyl are most prone to damage, but rigid ones can also eventually develop leaks.

Effect of static electricity

Rooms can be very dry, particularly in cold weather. If dry air conditions exist, and a film is pulled out quickly from the box or the cassette, friction usually occurs. This combination of friction and dry air produces static electricity. On the film, this static electricity appears as black electrostatic artifacts that look like lightening streaks, dots, starbursts or other shapes. These artifacts are more common on extraoral than on intraoral films. Therefore, darkrooms should be humidified during these periods and care should be taken in film handling throughout the entire process. The potential for development of static electricity exists any time until processing has begun.

Possible procedural errors

Light leaks in the darkroom can cause fogging or overexposure of a portion of the radiograph. Precautions against leakage are similar to those for other types of x-rays, but in addition the integrity of the film cassette should be checked as well. If the films are either under- or overexposed, the voltage and/or the current needs to be either increased or decreased respectively. Low developer solutions could cause underexposure as well. It is mandated that panoramic machines have markers distinguishing right from left on the image (typically "R" and "L"); if these are not visible on the radiograph, it should be thrown out. Patient identification should be done with a film imprinter or special tape or pen on the edge of the film after exposure and before processing, not incorporated before exposure. Double exposures should be discarded.

Panoramic tomography relative to intraoral radiographs

The area covered in a panoramic radiograph is much larger than combined intraoral techniques. Even in the full-mouth survey, intraoral radiographs basically cover the teeth, alveolar ridges, and some of the associated bone. Panoramic tomography extends the observed area far beyond these structures; the jaw, nasal cavities, and temporomandibular joint regions are now included increasing the diagnostic value. One newer diagnostic use is identification of calcifications in the carotid arteries, which if utilized in conjunction with other tests can help recognize stroke or other cerebrovascular risk Panoramic techniques

are generally easier and less time consuming than intraoral procedures, and therefore tend to cooperate more and the incidence of retakes is low. Radiation doses delivered during panoramic techniques are usually less than during other procedures, with the highest dose near the center of rotation.

Disadvantages of panoramic tomography relative to intraoral radiographs

Pantomograms generated during panoramic tomography tend to have a poorer image quality than intraoral radiographs. Use of intensifying screens or fast films with large grains further decreases this definition. In particular, the definition is decreased rendering panoramic radiography relatively unsuitable for certain diagnoses. Periodontal disease, tooth decay, and pathological conditions in the periapical region are not picked up well on pantomograms which means that bitewings and some periapical x-rays used in conjunction may be necessary. Only areas lying within the focal trough or image layer are distinct on panoramic radiographs, and machines with adjustable areas are expensive. In fact, any panoramic apparatus is generally costly. Lack of clarity can occur due to overlapping of images particularly in the premolar area, superimposition or obscuring of areas especially by the spinal column, and various sources of distortion. The panoramic machine should never be used in cases where only single or limited intraoral radiographs will suffice.

Guidelines for radiographic surveys in children

The best technique to use in children is a panoramic radiographic, if appropriate machinery is available, because it exposes them to less radiation. Posterior bitewings can be used supplementally. If a panoramic machine is unavailable, then the types of radiographs taken should depend on the child's age or dentition. Surveys for young children in the early eruptive stage (usually

- 136 -

up to 5 years of age) generally consist of occlusal films of both jaws and back apical and bitewing projections. Because their mouths are small, smaller No. 2 and No. 0 films are substituted instead of adult parameters. Between about 6 and 9 years of age, pediatric patients tend to have mixed dentition with both temporary and permanent teeth. In this age range, the radiographic documentation generally resembles a regular full-mouth survey except that smaller No. 1 films are usually used, with an occasional No. 2 film for posterior bitewings. Subjects in the older preadolescent group, about 10 to 12 years old, usually have a complete set of periapical films done.

Why radiographic surveys are important for pediatric subjects

Childhood is the time to diagnose and develop treatment plans for dental and other pathological problems. Dental cysts and tumors as well as other pediatric malignancies tend to occur during the period during childhood when teeth are developing. Children with genetic predisposition or other risk factors for caries should have posterior bitewings taken as soon as possible after the spaces between the teeth in these areas are closed up. If there is no decay, bitewings are generally done every year to 1 ½ years until permanent teeth come when the interval can be lengthened to 2 years.

Procedural parameters for periapical radiography in pediatric patients

The most important consideration when performing radiography on a pediatric patient is the reduction of radiation exposure. This reduction can be optimized by using a longer length positioning device, the higher potential difference range, the fastest film speed possible, a rectangular-shaped collimator, and a film holder that directs the beam. In addition, the child's body should be protected by lead shielding using both an apron for the torso region and a cervical

collar for the thyroid area. Child seats for positioning are also available.

Unique problems associated with endodontic radiography

Endodontic radiography is primarily used to look for dental pulp diseases. In this situation, the film is held in place by special film-holders and no bite block is used. A rubber barrier dam, hemostat, or other endodontic instruments are usually present in the oral cavity to facilitate visualization of the teeth and general area on the radiograph. These instruments will be visualized on the x-ray. Usually several different views are necessary to get a three-dimensional perspective. There are a number of commercially available endodontic film-holders. A hemostat also works quite well to hold the film in place using the paralleling technique, especially in the molar and pre-molar regions of the lower jaw. A number of views are usually documented, including from the top, from the back, and from the side.

Localizing entities like foreign objects on a radiograph

In general, there are two ways to localize entities like unerupted teeth, foreign bodies, or other irregularities on a radiograph. The first technique is the tube-shift method of localization in which a series of periapical radiographs is taken with the tubehead positioned differently horizontally for each. If the object in question shifts in harmony with the tubehead, it is located on the lingual or tongue side. If the entity appears to move in opposition to the tubehead, then it is located on the facial or buccal side. Another principle that can be applied to localization of objects is the buccal-object rule. Again two radiographs of a region are necessary; vertically aligned images are discriminated through changes in horizontal angulation of the x-ray beam while horizontal aligned images are discerned through changes in vertical angulation. Here hidden or unidentified entities that are buccal known objects move in the same direction as the x-ray beam or positioning device, and lingual objects shift in opposition to beam movement.

Documenting edentulous patients

Edentulous patients have partial or complete areas in their mouth where there are no teeth. A large proportion of these individuals have pathological abnormalities like infected areas, cysts, or remnants of roots or unerupted or extra teeth. If possible, a panoramic survey should be performed on edentulous individuals. Otherwise, a series of 10 to 14 different No. 2 periapical films is usually taken by directing the x-ray beam into the center of each film. Film-holders and the paralleling technique can be used in some of these patients without significant resorption. The bisecting angle method is also often used.

Radiographs and assessment of implant therapy

When sites for possible dental implants are selected, it is necessary to know the amount of bone present and the position of certain anatomical structures. Numerous images of the area are needed. Tomography should really be used to assess and obtain a three-dimensional view of various sites. Two different cuts, cross-sectional and sagittal, may be traced with linear tomography. Alternatively, computed tomography or a CT scan can be utilized. CT has some disadvantages including high cost, augmented radiation exposure, obscuration by artifacts, or general lack of image detail. In reality, many dental practices do not use tomography for assessment of implant therapy, substituting a combination of other types of radiographs. These substitutions are not recommended because they do not give accurate three-dimensional views.

Intensifying screens and extraoral radiography

Extraoral radiography is performed by resting a cassette along the side of the face or head and directing x-rays externally from the opposite side. Large screen films that are dual-coated with emulsion are inserted into the cassette which has intensifying screens on either side to form a sandwich. The intensifying screens serve to take in the radiation energy and convert it to light energy for latent image formation on the film. The intensifying screens have several layers for backing, support, and protection, but the most important layer is the phosphor layer. The phosphor layer contains a substance that will fluoresce or emit visible or other light when the x-ray strikes it. The film utilized should coordinate with the screen in terms of the spectral sensitivity or color range given off by the phosphor. The main purpose of intensifying screens is the amplification of the image which in turn reduces the necessary radiation dose.

Rare earth screen

A rare earth screen is an intensifying screen that incorporates elements as phosphors whose extraction from the earth is complex and costly. The spectral emission pattern of these elements, primarily lanthanum (La) and gadolinium (Gd) encompasses over half of the green wavelength area. Therefore, these types of screens are used in conjunction with films that have been developed to be sensitive to this green light spectrum area. One of the most widely used green-sensitive films is Kodak T-Mat film. T-Mat employs flat grains to increase the cross-sectional area, and it comes in several forms depending on the desired contrast.

Construction of extraoral cassettes

Extraoral cassettes are designed to enhance the penetration of the x-ray beam on the incoming side and stop the beam and its scatter on the far side. Therefore, the side placed against the patient is relatively thin and made of materials with small atomic numbers such as cardboard or plastic. The back is generally faced with a heavy metal like lead or aluminum. The film is layered between the two attached intensifying screens and held in place by some sort of device that applies pressure. There are usually external holding devices as well. Panoramic machines sometimes use a type of extraoral cassette that envelops a rotating drum apparatus; here the entire cassette must be more flexible and is generally made of plastic. Identification of the side of the patient and their name by some means is essential. Most of these cassettes have attachable lead pieces that say "R" or "L" for right or left.

Cephalometric radiography

Cephalometric radiography is a specialized technique that quantifies parameters of the skull in order to predict growth patterns. The method is used primarily by orthodontists or dentists that see mostly children. Cephalometric radiography requires a unique machine that employs an apparatus called a cephalostat to hold the individual's head in place with rods and ear posts. All measurements are made relative to the midsagittal or midline plane that divides the face in half, and the Frankfort line is used as the relative horizontal marker. The most popular stance is a lateral exposure with the cassette, located extraorally, against the left side of the face and the radiation beam projected a long way, about 5 feet, from the other side. The film must be placed in equidistant alignment to the midline. The radiograph is interpreted by looking at facial relationships and angles in an attempt to predict later growth patterns. Lateral oblique projections, where the beam is at a slight upward angle, are also done.

Posteroanterior projection

A posteroanterior projection is an extraoral exposure of the skull taken by directing the x-ray beam from about 3 feet behind the patient. The central ray is aimed at the occipital protuberance in the ear, and the film is in front of the individual normally with the forehead and nose positioned against the cassette. This technique is useful for identification of fractures, malignancies, and widespread disease states in the skull area. A variation in which the patient opens their mouth and places their chin and nose against the cassette is called the Waters' view. This change enables visualization of the middle of the face, in particular the maxillary sinus region.

Projections taken to observe the TMJ region

The TMJ or temporomandibular joint connects the mandible to the temporal bone on the side of the head. Visualization of this region is diagnostic for a number of problems. The radiographic techniques are very specialized and generally are performed outside the normal dental practice. In a normal dental office, the only types of TMJ analysis usually available are either transcranial lateral projections are specialized adaptations of panoramic projections. A transcranial lateral view obliquely angles the center of the x-ray beam from above toward the condyle on the opposing side; the image is usually quite distorted and does not pick up some vital diagnostic areas. Specialized panoramic projections can be used to pick up obvious changes, but the beam can only be directed obliquely to the axis of the condyle which limits the utility of this technique as well. Sometimes submentovertex projections, where the beam is directed from below the chin, are used to observe TMJ.

How TMJ tomography is performed

The TMJ region is usually documented in specialized facilities that have machines to perform analysis beyond the usual projections. One of the techniques used for

TMJ is TMJ tomography. The principle involved is similar to panoramic radiography in that an x-ray tube and film cassette are rotating in opposite directions around a central fixed point in this case. The focal plane is primarily visualized and the rest is blurry. The thickness of the focal plane is controlled by the angle between shots, and its position is influenced by the position of the central fulcrum. The relationship between the tube and film can be either linear or in some other trajectory like circular, elliptical, or cloverleaf. CT scanning is a type of tomography that uses digital imagery; the method is more expensive but can provide finer details.

Magnetic resonance imaging used to analyze the TMJ region

Magnetic resonance imaging or MRI can be employed to visualize the TMJ or other areas without the use of ionizing radiation. It is the only technique that can document all areas related to TMJ functional abnormalities, including the discs and rear attachments of the temporomandibular joints, the condyle and the fossae or groove of the lower jaw. In MRI, the individual is subjected to a magnetic field. Atoms of hydrogen in the body are realigned by the electromagnetic forces generated. After the area being documented is subsequently bombarded with radio frequency waves, the protons release the energy absorbed. A sensor picks up this information and sends it to a computer which provides an image. The technique is especially useful for visualization of soft tissues.

Types of CT scans

CT or computed tomography scans are images produced by directing an x-ray beam at an individual and then digitally transmitting information about the degree of penetration to electronic sensors. The number of pixels in an area is directly related to the density of the tissue, and they are represented as CT numbers or Hounsfield units. Tissue types have characteristic units; for example, water has 0 Hounsfield units, while bone has +1000 and air has -1000 units. No film is utilized as in other forms of tomography. The beam is projected through the patient while rotating through a plane. This plane can be axial, coronal or sagittal meaning it is either parallel to the ground, through the imaginary line dividing the front and back of the head, or through the midline separating right and left. Some CT scanners, in particular those used for the head and neck region, project a beam that is either round or cone-shaped onto a two-dimensional detector. In this case, radiation exposure is minimized.

Advantages and disadvantages of computed tomography

Computed tomography is great at distinguishing between slight differences in tissue density, and in addition contrast and density can be manipulated to look at different areas. CT can be done in a variety of planes while eliminating superimposition of unnecessary images outside the focal plane. Pictures can be reformatted relative to other planes. The technique is easy and accurate. However, the patient is generally exposed to more radiation with CT than with ordinary film techniques, although dosage can be reduced through use of cone beam machines or software that localizes the imaging. The latter is often used for dental implant preparation. Considerably more radiation is delivered during CT scanning of the head than an ordinary skull film, but this negative aspect is obliterated by the high incidence of repeats in skull filming. CT scans are more costly to the patient than films. Metals in the field produce CT scan artifacts just as they do on films.

When a digital image is generated

Digitization is the transformation of pieces of an analog image into relative intensities and the reassembly of these intensities into a visible analog image on a computer screen.

An ordinary radiograph is an analog image because the finished product is a direct representation of what has been documented on film. Digital procedures take the analog image and initially convert it to numbers on a grid that represent relative levels of brightness. The number within each grid measures the number of pixels or tiny dots of light in that area. No film or processing is required with digital imaging, the radiation dose is low, and the cost is minimal. The computer-generated images can be viewed right away, manipulated, or transmitted electronically. Use of digital imaging is controversial, however, because it does not produce a hard copy and it may not be recognized legally or by insurance companies. Initial cost outlay is considerable and the quality of the image is generally inferior to film techniques.

Spatial resolution on a digital image

The spatial resolution of a digital image is the relative ability to differentiate line pairs on it. The property is quantified in terms of line pairs observable per millimeter. Line pairs and pixels or dots of light are both directly related to the clarity or spatial resolution of the image. Humans can usually only differentiate about 12 to 14 line pairs (lp) per millimeter (mm). If the pixel size is decreased, more pixels and therefore more line pairs can fit in a space. The maximal levels of spatial resolution for intraoral detectors are currently 20 lp/mm, which is better than what human beings can resolve.

Gray scale resolution on a digital image

Gray scale resolution is the total number of shades of gray that a particular digital image is capable of displaying. Every pixel in the image has an assigned number which is related to the computer storage capacity. Each bit of computer storage capacity exponentially increases the gray scale resolution according to the formula 2^x with x = number of bits of storage capacity. While current computers may have up to 12 bits or more of storage space, 8 bits are shown on the monitor generally. Since 8 bits represents 2^8 or 256 shades of gray, considerably more than can be distinguished by the human eye, this is sufficient. The numbering is represented as 0 for pure black up to 255 for pure white.

Selection of a computer to perform digital imaging

At present only personnel computers or PCs with Windows capability can interface with digital imaging software. Either a laptop or desktop model can be used. The processor speed determines the rapidity of image processing; at least 266 MHz should be selected. Sufficient random access memory or RAM should be chosen to enable data retention and processing during the exposure without having to temporary store the information on the hard drive; this means that generally the minimum RAM should be 64 megabytes. After processing, the image probably will be kept on the hard drive so its memory should be large, at least about 15 gigabytes. Various types of printers, each with its own pros and cons, can be selected. A laptop comes with an integrated monitor, but the screen may not offer the contrast or intensity of other options. Regular cathode ray tube (CRT) monitors display the image very nicely but are heavy, whereas a flat screen is thinner and offers excellent image quality. A number of dental imaging software packages are available; it is preferable to buy one that conforms to standards established by Digital Imaging and Communication in Medicine or DICOM.

Equipment and procedures required to acquire digital imagery

Regular radiographic films can be converted to digital images, a process known as the indirect method of obtaining a digital image. In this technique, some type of camera or scanner is used. In the first case, a digital or video camera takes a picture of an extant radiograph. If a video camera is used, a

- 141 -

computer transforms the image into a digital one. If a digital camera is utilized, the digitization occurs internally and the picture is later downloaded onto a computer. Indirect acquisition can also be done with a scanner with an attached transparency adaptor that delivers light through the x-ray. This light is then transmitted to a chip known as a charge coupled device or CCD which assembles a digital image.

Charge coupled device

A charge coupled device or CCD is one type of sensor that can detect x-rays and transform them into electronic data for computer interpretation and visualization. CCDs consist of transistor grids that change x-ray photons striking them into electrons. CCDs can be used with visible light. For x-ray exposures, the beam passes through a scintillation screen and a fiber-optic faceplate before reaching the CCD sensor. The scintillation screen serves to convert the x-ray picture into fluorescing visible light. The fiber-optic plate focuses the light and reduces passage of the x-rays by use of leaded glass. The charge coupled device receives the light as pixels on the grid, which are then interpreted in terms of brightness and position to form a digital image. CCDs are used in direct digital imaging or indirectly in conjunction with a scanner.

CMOS/APS

CMOS/APS is the abbreviation for a Complementary Metal Oxide Semiconductor with an Active Pixel Sensor. It is another device used to directly produce digital images from x-ray exposure. It is similar to a charge coupled device in that it employs a scintillation screen to convert the x-rays to visible light and an integrated circuit board to convert the light to digital images for computer interpretation. The main difference between CMOS/APS devices and CCDs is that the CMOS/APS includes amplifying transistors on each of the pixels. Advantages of CMOS/APS sensors include the ability to put circuitry directly onto the chip, use of less power, and reduction of pixel size. These devices can also be linked to a computer via a simple USB port.

Photostimulable phosphor imaging

Photostimulable phosphor (PSP) imaging is one method of converting x-ray exposures directly into digital images. Rare earth phosphors, typically barium europium fluorohalide, are coated onto imaging plates. When x-rays strike these plates, the radiation energy is amassed on the plate as a type of latent image until processing. PSP plates are later processed by scanning them with a laser to produce fluorescence. The signals are interpreted by a photodiode which transfers the digital image to a computer. PSP imaging uses plates that are similar in size to regular dental films. Other advantages of this system include less radiation to the patient, an expanded and linear range of exposures that can produce a good image, and the ability to take the film without being hooked up to a computer.

Digital image sensors and the computer

Charge coupled devices (CCDs) currently interface with the computer for digital imaging via a Universal Serial Bus (USB) or Firewall connector. Older CCD sensor systems utilize computers with special circuit boards incorporated into them, but newer models can process the picture through external packs or processing boards. CMOS/APS sensors generally interface with the computer through a simple USB port. Both CCD and CMOS sensors produce images on the computer within seconds. PSP plates do not directly connect to the computer; instead the laser scanner (which fluoresces the latent image on the plate) is directly attached to the computer. The time between exposure and reading for PSP imaging is much longer than that required with the other sensors.

Digital imaging and panoramic or cephalometric machinery

Charge coupled devices and photostimulable phosphor systems are both currently used with many panoramic or cephalometric systems. For PSP systems, the major adaptations are larger plates and scanners to accommodate the cassette. Resolution in terms of line pairs per millimeter is generally reduced for PSP relative to regular films when panoramic views are taken in order to reduce scan time and film size. On the other hand, CCD sensors can be used at resolutions comparable to regular film for panoramic or cephalometric views. These types of machines used multiple CCD devices stacked into a grid-like linear array. The array travels around or scans the individual gathering a series of single vertical lines to form the image. Most new CCD panoramic systems do only digital imaging, but there are kits available that convert film-based machines for digital use.

Infection control procedures

None of the detectors used with digital processes can be sterilized using heat, and cold chemical methods of sterilization are impractical as well. Infection control procedures for digital imaging with charge coupled devices or CMOS sensors are similar. For both, two layers of plastic barriers are used, a sleeve and an additional finger wrapper. For phosphor (PSP) apparatuses, the primary infection control procedure is the placement of the plate in some type of commercially-available barrier envelope before exposure. The plate is kept bagged until before it is placed in the scanner.

CMOS or CCD sensors and film-based systems

Detectors used for CMOS or CCD digital imaging are thicker than normal film. This difference means that either film-holders must be converted to accommodate the sensors or proprietary holders must be utilized. After positioning, the software in the computer regulates the sensor and clarifies the appropriate time to snap the exposure. Since no development is necessary for either of these techniques, the image is available within seconds, and the viewpoint or characteristics of the picture can be modified with the software.

Steps involved in PSP digital imaging

For digital imaging that utilizes photostimulable phosphors, the first step is the erasure of images on the plates from previous exposures. This step is very easy. Basically, the phosphor-coated side of the plate is set on top of a lighted viewbox for several minutes to obliterate the prior image. Then the plates are enclosed in tight barrier envelopes or the panoramic cassette. The x-ray exposure is taken. Then the covering is removed, and the PSPs are loaded onto a drum. This drum is placed into the scanner, and the exposures are scanned with a laser. The images are transmitted directly to a computer.

Modifications using digital imaging processing

Various software and other tools incorporated into digital imaging processing equipment can be used to modify the image for better visualization or diagnostic purposes. One of the most common software packages can turn over the generated picture to give the mirror image; this is used to orient the views like a conventional film array. There are various controls that can change the brightness, manipulate the contrast into a suitable gray scale range, or zoom for magnification of specific areas. There is usually a mechanism to exchange black and white areas or reverse the gray scale in order to see certain objects better, and another that colorizes or designates a color to the gray ratio. The computer usually has incorporated filters to reduce noise and sharpen the picture. Software may also permit measurement of certain areas on the film.

Subtraction radiography

Subtraction radiography is a technique employed with digital image processing. The technique digitally merges two different images and then subtracts the common areas from the radiographic representation. Therefore, only the variations between the original images are seen. This practice is useful for visualization of sequential changes in decay development or bone loss as well as for observation after surgical procedures such as implants or periodontia. At present, the legal implications of permanent storage of this type of manipulation of the images as well as other modifications are somewhat unresolved. Usually the manipulated image can only be earmarked as a copy, not an original.

Storage of digital radiographic images

Original or manipulated images can be stored on the computer with software that typically compresses or reduces the size of the file. Files can be compressed with either no loss of computer data or with some ("lossy") deficit of original data. Both methods permanently change the image, but studies have found that diagnostic utility is not compromised with compression up to 1/12 of the original. Digital image formats include TIFF, which does not discard any data, and JPEG, which does reduce the image as much as 100 times and is therefore a lossy compression. Thus the JPEG format can initiate image degradation. Typically, the images are also backed-up onto CD-ROMs, DVD-ROMs, or various forms of magnetic digital tapes. They can also be transmitted via networking to other individuals.

Structures on radiographs are generally interpreted

Teeth and other structures or areas on a radiograph are generally interpreted in terms of how radiolucent or radiopaque they are. Radiolucent areas allow a great deal of radiation to penetrate them and thus appear dark or black on the radiograph. Radiopaque areas block the passage of x-rays and thus emerge as relatively light or white on the radiographic image. These terms are used not only for film-based radiographs, but also to describe the relative densities generated using other techniques such as computed tomography. Radiopaque sections are described as being denser than radiolucent portions. These known density differences are used to interpret the structures and processes observed on the radiograph or a computer-generated image.

Areas in the mouth that are radiopaque

The enamel of the teeth, the dentin underneath, and another part called the lamina dura all appear as white or somewhat light areas on a radiograph. These structures all absorb the x-rays to some extent. The enamel or hard calcium-containing layer on the outside of the tooth is very white on a radiograph, while the underlying dentin is slightly less dense and appears lighter on the image. Tooth decay or caries can be visualized in both these areas. There is also a very delicate layer of alveolar bone surrounding the tooth socket called the lamina dura which also should be radiopaque on the radiograph. This bone becomes thicker at the top when a new tooth is emerging, and it can shrivel or disappear in certain disease states. The other portions of the alveolar bone surround the teeth and are relatively radiopaque as well. Thinning of this bone suggests a disease state such as periodontal disease or even osteoporosis.

Areas in the mouth that are radiolucent

There is a cavity enclosed by the dentin and enamel of the tooth called the pulp space. This cavity is radiolucent or dark on a radiograph generally. The portion protruding down into the apex of the root of the tooth is termed the root canal space and it should appear radiolucent on the image as well. The pulp areas can become inflamed secondary to microbial infections from injury or diseases of the teeth or surrounding areas. Typically, there is also a dark or radiolucent border between the lamina dura and the root section of the teeth representing the periodontal ligament space (PDLS). This space appears wider in a number of metastatic diseases or if the teeth have been shifted (primarily through orthodontia).

Anatomical structures that appear radiolucent

The anatomical structures of the maxilla or upper jaw that appear radiolucent on a radiograph are those that are some type of natural opening or groove. One of these structures is the median maxillary or palatal suture. This structure is a fixed joint in the roof of the mouth beginning at the center of the incisors and extending posterior along the midline. There is also a dark cavity to either side of the front of this line called the nasopalatine or incisive foramen, whose major function is to receive nerve responses and blood vessels. Occasionally, four cavities are observed instead of two. If the area has a white border, cyst formation is suggested. Any hollows containing air are dark-appearing nasal fossae, including small indentations in the alveolar bone of either jaw called incisive lateral fossae. These areas do not indicate disease processes. Parts of the maxillary sinus appear radiolucent as well.

Maxillary sinus on a radiograph

The maxillary sinus or antrum is a hollow space within the alveolar bone that contains air. It is one of the sinuses surrounding the nose. Typically, only the bottom half of this cavity is observed on a periapical projection as a radiolucent shadow surrounded by a delicate jagged radiopaque edge. Occasionally, this sinus cavity will expand into the area between the roots of the back teeth and form what looks like a depression. This condition is referred to as pneumatization, and it can be observed with

chronic sinus diseases, aging, or early extraction of molars in the maxillary jaw.

Anatomical structures that appear radiopaque

There are several characteristic anatomical structures in the maxilla that appear radiopaque or relatively white on a radiograph. Typically, a white section that looks like an inverted Y is seen in the canine area. This inverted Y represents the junction between front border of the maxillary sinus and the floor of the nasal fossa. The area is used as a landmark even in toothless individuals, and pathological conditions can change its appearance. Tuberosities are rounded protruberances found in the back of the jaw; they also are relatively radiopaque. Just behind the tuberosity, another light area called the hamular process can be seen; it resembles a hook. One of the cheek bones in the upper jaw is termed the zygomatic or malar bone, and it is generally visualized as a radiopaque U-shaped area or arch above the teeth.

Anatomical structures that appear radiopaque

The coronoid process is the forward-sloping triangular shaped portion of the mandible or lower jaw. It projects from the sigmoid notch of the mandible and connects to a muscle called the temporalis. This process appears relatively radiopaque on a radiograph, and it is often seen on images of the maxilla because of its proximity. Other radiopaque areas in the front of the mandible include the mental ridges or bones on the front of the lower jaw, parts of the genial tubercles below and along the midline, and the lower cortex of the jaw. White lines are also seen extending from the mental tubercle back to the anterior portion of the branching ramus (the external oblique ridge) and lingually from the pre-molar to molar regions (mylohyoid line). The softer tissues are sometimes seen as relatively radiopaque areas on the image if pressure from biting the film packet forces them into the area being x-rayed.

Anatomical structures that appear radiolucent

In the front of the mandible, there are two radiolucent areas. The first is the mental foramen, which is a round-shaped section just below both sets of pre-molars; its serves as a tributary for nerve impulses and blood vessels. There is a genial tubercle along the midline in the front of mandible, which appears as a dark spot in the middle for passage of blood vessels surrounded by a lighter area where muscles are attached. There is also a dark passage called the mandibular or inferior alveolar canal that runs down the side of the lower jaw between the mandibular foramen and the mental foramen; a major artery traces the canal area and relatively light areas are seen to either side.

Endodontic and other restorative materials

Various types of foreign restorative materials are inserted into the dental cavity for treatment of endodontic or pulp diseases. These materials can contain silver, gold, a pliable latex substance called gutta percha, or various amalgams (typically mercury, silver, and tin). During the actual endodontic process, other objects like rubber clamps or files might be inserted into the region as well. On a radiograph, all of these materials are observed as intensely radiopaque, even relative to the tooth enamel. Other restorative materials that appear radiopaque can include newer tooth-colored composites and various types of cements. On the other hand, many modern restorations utilize acrylic or composites made with it, and the acrylic is radiolucent. Older porcelain crowns also appear relatively dark on the image.

Orthodontic devices, pediatric restorations, and prosthodontic materials

Most orthodontic devices are bands, wires, brackets, spacers or retainers containing stainless steel, and therefore they are seen as intensely radiopaque areas on radiographs. Unfortunately, some of these devices obscure evidence of underlying tooth decay. There are also newer clear plastic aligners available, but these would normally be removed before the shot. Prosthodontic materials like dentures or bridges should also be taken out before radiographs are taken. Again these devices mask other disease processes if left in; the metallic portions would appear extremely white and the porcelain or acrylic sections would prevent absorption of the radiation and seem darker. Infrequently, materials inserted for hygienic or periodontal purposes may also show up as radiopaque areas on an image.

Radiographic appearance of foreign materials inserted during oral surgery

There are a variety of wires, bars, crowns, bridges, and screws that might be permanently or temporarily inserted into the jaw area during oral surgery. Usually these insertions are done after some sort of traumatic incident like an automobile accident or explosion. Most of the foreign materials utilized contain a metal, either stainless steel or some type of amalgam, which means that they appear as very white, radiopaque areas on the radiograph. Bone should abut the implant. White fragments visualized on an image can also be clues to a patient's history, because these pieces can remain imbedded.

Foreign materials that might be seen on a radiograph

Sometimes devices used during the exposure of a radiograph might appear on the image. For example, biteblocks are often seen as either white regions (if metallic) or relatively dark areas (if plastic). Other devices used to position the film can be seen as radiopaque areas, and there are varieties of previously described artifacts with characteristic appearances. External jewelry, eyeglasses or other materials are generally observed as white areas. In addition, occasionally radiopaque materials are injected into various passages to visualize structures or make them denser; these areas will be light on the radiograph as well.

Periodontal disease

Periodontal disease is a blanket term for processes that change the gums or tissues that envelop and support the teeth. The majority of these diseases are caused by microbial infections resulting from plaque buildup, other pathogenic exposure, restorative work, or tartar. The disease is distinguished by inflamed gums, development of pockets in the area, and damage to the associated ligaments and alveolar bone. Progression of bone loss is diagnostic for periodontitis. Periodontal pockets are grooves of soft tissue that can be identified only by use of probing instruments. If left untreated, periodontal disease can result in tooth loss.

Sequential radiographs for diagnosis of periodontal disease

Radiographs cannot show depth, and thus bones and teeth are generally visually laid over each other in the image. This means that a single radiograph might pick up bone loss and indicate periodontal disease, but it is not useful in determining the extent or rate of progression of the condition. Small amounts of bone loss are difficult to see on an individual image. On the other hand, if sequential radiographs at different time intervals are taken, changes can be visualized using computerized digital subtraction. The two images are digitally merged, the common areas are subtracted out, and the resultant picture shows only the differences. Tiny changes can be measured by this technique.

The paralleling method with high voltage and a long positioning device should be used.

Methods used to diagnose periodontal disease

Periodontal disease is diagnosed by a combination of methods. Pockets are generally identified by probing with an instrument or by inserting radiopaque substances in the area and taking an exposure. Visualization of bone requires sequential radiography and digital subtraction techniques. Radiographs alone cannot determine the characteristics of the bone deformity. There is also an instrument called the Nabors probe that can be used to detect furcation or separation of the tooth from the underlying bone; sometimes this can be seen radiographically as a dark area. Dental calculus or mineralization can sometimes be picked up as white lines or spurs on exposures. Progression toward tooth loosening can be diagnosed if the periodontal ligament space gets wider, but this is rarely observable on a radiograph because other structures obscure the changes.

Changes associated with periodontal disease seen on a radiograph

An early radiographic indication of periodontal disease is the blurring or discontinuity of the lamina dura or bone surrounding the periodontal ligament. These are known as irregularities of the alveolar bone crest. Another early indication is the widening of the periodontal ligament space which can sometimes be seen as a darker triangular or funnel-like area. Radiographs can sometimes pick up early interseptal bone changes as dark protrusions into the alveolar bone region. The mechanism involved is the expansion of blood vessels in the bone as a result of increased inflammation of the gum. The concentration of minerals in the tissues is decreased as well. Eventually, the teeth may appear to be completely detached from the underlying bone. Calculus deposits may be seen between the surfaces of the teeth.

Determining bone loss by observation of a radiograph

Bone loss is actually evaluated by comparing the amount of enduring bone to the expected amount of bone. The most common site for initial evaluation is the interproximal septal bone. The cementoenamel junction (CEJ) is the part of the tooth where the enamel ends and the dentin starts. The distance from that point towards the apex of the tooth is normally 1 to 1.5 millimeters; therefore bone loss is measured as the difference between the observed height and the expected height. Bone loss can be generalized (evident consistently on the majority of teeth), or it can be localized to only certain teeth. In either case, inflammatory processes resulting from periodontitis usually occur concurrently, and thus loss of contact between the dentition is also observed on the radiograph.

Bone loss observed on a radiograph

Bone loss can occur in different planes. If the deficiency is generally found in plane equidistant from the CEJ of adjoining teeth, the loss is considered horizontal. If the pattern of bone loss is more angular and inconsistent between adjacent teeth, the loss is defined as vertical or angular. The latter configuration may also show enlargement of the periodontal ligament space or pockets below the bone. Both types of bone loss probably involve local inflammatory responses, but a vertical pattern may indicate systemic involvement as well. Evidence of vertical bone loss without accompanying plaque buildup or gingivitis in teenagers is called localized juvenile periodontitis or LJP. LJP often occurs in the premolar-molar region and the rate of bone loss can be very high. The etiology of LPJ is unclear, but it probably infectious or immunologic in nature.

Landmarks used to determine bone height

The level of bone on the facial side can be estimated by using the lamina dura. The lamina dura is the portion of the bone using seen as a radiopaque line on the radiograph. The point at which it starts to become less opaque or solid is a good approximation of where the interseptal bone begins. The level of bone on the lingual or tongue side is usually determined by finding the faint line that undulates across the center of the teeth. This line distinguishes between the areas of the root that are covered by bone and those that are not and represents the level of the alveolar crest. From the alveolar crest to the apex is the bone height for the lingual aspect.

Infrabony pockets

Infrabony pockets are regions created through crestal bone loss and observed on radiographs as dark areas protruding into the bone area between the teeth. These pockets or defects are classified according to the number of bony walls forming the area, typically one-, two-, three-, or four-walled. A one-wall or hemiseptum defect occurs when only one wall of the interseptal bone is damaged leaving the other intact. Two-wall infrabony pockets are the most common type, in particular a variant called an osseous crater which constitutes over half of all defects in the lower jaw. An osseous crater appears on the radiograph as a concave indentation in the bone between two teeth. A three-wall pocket is bounded by three bony walls and the root, and a four-wall defect entirely encompasses the root area. Usually these defects are confirmed by probing with an instrument.

Furcation involvement

Teeth further back in the jaw can be bifurcated or trifurcated. In other words, they can have roots that branch or divide into two parts or three parts because the periodontal pocket has enlarged. If there is a pocket in the gum tissue around the root, there is furcation involvement. A radiograph that shows widening of the periodontal ligament space or significant bone loss suggests furcation. Usually, the dentist investigates this condition by inserting a probe into the top of the area (possibly in conjunction with warm condensed air). Furcation involvement can be found near many teeth, but it is observed most often initially in the first molar area.

Causes that can predispose an individual

Periodontal disease is primarily an inflammatory disease of the gum area caused by buildup of bacterial plaque. There are a number of factors that can bias an individual toward development of this buildup. A radiograph can only detect these factors; it cannot determine the exact role they may play in development of periodontal disease. The first element is deposition of calculus or tartar, which is the concretion of bacteria and other organic materials on the surface of the tooth. Calculus is often described in terms of where it is found and the source of the other organic materials; supragingival and subgingival calculus have contributions from saliva and serum respectively. Restorations or implants that are done incorrectly are other significant causes of periodontal disease because they can leave overhangs or gaps where bacteria can grow and attach. Similarly, areas that allow food to become impacted or stuck can predispose a person to periodontal disease. Examples of these types of areas include sections that have worn away on the tooth surface or are decayed.

Functional problems that contribute to periodontal disease

The two most common functional issues that contribute to periodontal disease development are occlusal traumatism and a high crown-to-root ratio. The occlusal surfaces of the teeth can become traumatized primarily through undesirable oral practices such as grinding of the teeth (known as bruxism) or firmly holding and clenching the teeth. These practices tend to collapse the underlying ligaments, cause bone to reabsorb, enlarge the periodontal ligament space, and eventually lead to loosening of the teeth. Radiographs can aid with clinical diagnosis of occlusal traumatism. In addition, when individuals have teeth with long crowns relative to the root, or a high crown-to-root ratio, the load applied to the gum is high. This condition can be clearly seen on a radiograph, and it is prevalent in the Latin American population.

Radiographs used to determine periodontal damage

Periodontal damage can be an active or relatively static process, and radiographs are useful for determination of the rate of destruction of the gum area. The appearance of the crests of the interseptal alveolar bone is generally used to assess the activity level. If this crest is uneven and less well-defined, the periodontal destruction is probably active. If on the other hand, the crest is smooth, distinct, and relatively radiopaque, the gingival breakdown is not active at that time. Usually diagnosis is made by comparing sequential radiographs. The prognosis or final outcome can be only be estimated by assimilation of all available data, which should include radiographs and clinical evaluation.

Dental caries

Dental caries or tooth decay is the breakdown of hard dentin tissue in a tooth. Caries development is dependent on three aspects. All must be present for tooth decay to occur. First, the host must have a propensity towards caries development. Then, specific bacteria or microflora must be present. Lastly, dietary sugars that can ferment or be broken down into acids and other substances must be available. The acids are the substances that actually demineralize or decalcify and break down the hard enamel of the tooth. As the breakdown proceeds over time, eventually tooth decay or caries can be detected. Typically, radiographic visualization occurs when about half the calcium and phosphorus is broken down.

Interproximal enamel caries and its characteristic radiographic appearance

Interproximal enamel caries is the tooth decay that occurs between two abutting tooth surfaces. Initially, interproximal enamel caries starts just underneath the point of contact; at this point, the lesion looks white and chalky and a small dark notch is visible on a radiograph. As the destruction proceeds, the shape of the lesion usually becomes an elongated triangle. The longer tip of the triangle is directed downward toward the dentinoenamel junction (DEJ). Caries visualization on a radiograph is influenced by the spatial parameters of the adjoining tooth, in particular the area of the contact point which can obscure the extent of the decay.

Incipient, lamellar, and dentinal caries

There are several types of interproximal enamel caries that do not have the characteristic triangular appearance running along the edge of the tooth. One is incipient caries, which is decay that has not completely penetrated the enamel. On a radiograph, incipient caries usually looks like ca small, dark funnel-shaped area. Another type is lamellar caries, which appears as a dark line that progresses into the dentin region. There can also be decay primarily within the dentin called dentinal caries. This type of decay looks restricted to areas under the enamel on a radiograph, and it can destroy tubules in the dentin.

Radiographic classification system for dental caries

The extent of dental caries is currently classified into 4 groups depending on the penetration of the destruction as visualized on a radiograph. The decision to treat caries should be based upon the combination of this radiographic classification and clinical evaluation. For both C-1 and C-2 radiographic caries, only the enamel is penetrated, and the major difference between the two is the degree of penetration (less than half-way for C-1, half-way or greater for C-2). If there is some infiltration of the dentin area as well, the caries is classified as C-3 or C-4. C-3 means less than half the dentin has been penetrated and C-4 indicates deeper decay.

Acute versus chronic caries and rampant caries

The terms acute and chronic as applied to dental caries differentiate between the rates of penetration of the lesion, in other words fast versus slower. In addition acute caries tends to arise from a relatively tiny surface point compared to chronic cases. Tooth decay in younger people tends to proceed more rapidly than in older individuals. For example, a condition called rampant caries, in which the decay has an abrupt onset and extremely rapid progression, commonly occurs only in children and adolescents. Rampant caries is rarely found in adults, except in some cases of xerostomia or dry mouth. Acute caries is prevalent from adolescence to about age 25, and chronic tooth decay is usually the type found above that age range.

Clinical progression and radiographic appearance of occlusal caries

Caries that begins on the occlusal surface of a tooth is extremely common in younger patients, particularly in the molar and pre-molar regions. The occlusal surfaces of teeth in these areas are very uneven and layered deeply with enamel. Poor dental hygiene in the back of the mouth increases the possibility of caries in this area. The tooth decay is usually not detected on a radiograph until it has broken through the dentinoenamel junction, at which point it appears as a dark line or region just below the DEJ. Actually the caries spreads up into the enamel as well. Therefore, mirrors and certain probes are usually used to identify cases of occlusal caries.

Radiographic appearance of caries on the facial or lingual sides of the tooth

Tooth decay can occur on the facial or lingual sides of the tooth as well as the neck or cervical region of the crown. The point of entrance of the caries is usually relatively large compared to other decay types. These types of lesions are visualized as very well-defined radiolucent circular areas on the radiograph generally, although they might also appear as dark oval or arc shapes. Caries on these surfaces is hard to detect until it has progressed to a certain point. These smooth surface types of caries are usually identified by using a mirror and some type of exploratory probe.

Diagnostic value of radiographs in assessment of pulpal caries

A radiograph is of limited value in the diagnostic evaluation of pulpal caries. Pulpal caries is decay that has extended into the central tooth pulp which contains nerve endings and blood vessels. Since radiographs cannot show depth, it is very difficult to angle the beam to pick up pulp involvement without creating other distortions. In particular, the exposure may obscure the extent or absence of pulpal involvement because the radiolucent decay area is shown over the pulp. This distortion is exaggerated further if the picture is overexposed.

Causes and radiographic appearance of root caries

Tooth decay can occur in the root area of the tooth without enamel involvement. This type of root or cemental caries usually begins in the cementoenamel junction or CEJ region as a result of plaque retention along receding gums. The caries usually radiates outward from the point of origin eventually merging into a circular area. Radiographically the decay appears to engulf and blur the entire

root area, and clinically it erodes the cementum located at the CEJ. The enamel is not directly affected, but cemental caries can broaden into regions very close to it. Root caries is prevalent in the elderly population.

Causes and appearance of secondary caries

Secondary caries is tooth decay that emerges after restorations for various types of previous caries. It is usually visualized on a radiograph as a dark radiolucent spot near the restoration. The secondary or recurrent caries can have two different types of causes. In some cases, dentitional caries in the hard part of the tooth under the enamel was not entirely eradicated before the restoration was done. New caries can also develop if tin or zinc leaks out from the filling or cement. In the latter case, the current theory is that the metal ions combine with demineralized dentin to initiate fresh areas of decay.

Theories about caries that have been halted

Various types of caries can be halted or arrested if the environmental milieu changes into one that does not promote decay. Incipient caries, in which the decay has not penetrated much of the enamel, is common, and typically the enamel is as hard as that in a healthy tooth. The mechanism in this case is probably remineralization of the enamel. This type of arrested caries is often seen adjacent to another tooth that has been removed. Sometimes tooth decay on occlusal surfaces stops because the dentin has become so hard upon repeated buffing that bacteria are sloughed off. In this case, there is a characteristic radiographic appearance including a missing crown with a ragged, radiolucent space in its place.

Reasons the extent of caries can be overlooked

The relative thickness of the tooth and its area of decay can influence interpretation of the extent of caries on a radiograph. X-ray beams are impeded and absorbed by interaction with the enamel. In areas where the carious lesion is narrowing, such as where it may be entering the dentin, the large enamel area can obscure the much smaller radiolucent decay area. In addition, at least half the calcium and phosphorus must be destroyed before a lesion can be visualized on a radiograph, a trait that leads to inherent underestimation of caries involvement.

Cervical burnout

Cervical burnout is an artifact that appears to be caries on an exposure. The cervical neck of the tooth is tapered. Therefore it attracts fewer energy photons and appears darker on a radiograph than the crown above or root below it. Thus a radiolucent band or collar may be observed on a radiograph, but there is actually no decay. In the posterior teeth, the radiographic appearance of cervical burnout can be more pie-shaped. Similar contrast artifacts may be observed at the cementoenamel junction, with certain root arrangements, or if the beam is directed incorrectly horizontally. Correct horizontal angulation usually eliminates cervical burnout.

Restorative materials that resemble caries formation

Restorative dental materials made from substances that are also radiolucent like decay can resemble caries formation on a radiograph. In general, this situation only occurs when the restoration is relatively old and materials like certain plastics, silicates, or calcium hydroxide were used. The cements used to affix these materials generally contain metals, however; the adjacent cement appears as a white area on the exposure therefore and aids in differentiation between these materials and true decay. Newer restorations generally are comprised of high molecular weight metals, either gold or amalgam mixtures rendering them radiopaque. Thus newer dental work is rarely confused with caries.

Tooth enamel and caries on a radiograph

Areas of the tooth can be mechanically worn down and look like caries on a radiograph. One type of corrosion is called attrition, in which occlusal or incisal edges are worn down. If the attrition is severe enough to include dentin involvement, a hollow space that appears to be caries can develop. The other type of corrosion that mimics decay is called abrasion, and it is usually observed in the root area with receding gums. In addition, there is a condition called enamel hypoplasia in which incomplete development results in fissures in the enamel. These fissures may stain and appear to be decay. Enamel hypoplasia can be distinguished from caries by using an exploratory probe; the probe detaches easily in hypoplasia but does not with true caries.

Periapical disease

Periapical disease is any disruption of the lamina dura at the apex of a tooth. The lamina dura is the cortical bone surrounding the periodontal ligament. Healthy individuals have dense lamina dura that appear radiographically as a narrow, white line running near the apex of the tooth. When the line loses its continuous appearance due to resorption of the lamina dura and alveolar bone, some sort of periapical disease exists. The classification of the type of periapical disease generally requires additional clinical investigation. Some periapical diseases are acutely symptomatic with pain and edema, but others persist chronically without significant clinical signs. Many of these conditions are actually periodontal disease as well.

Pulp area development and pulpitis

The pulp chamber and its canal are areas in the middle of the crown and root of the tooth. Generally, they do not contain calcified materials like bones do, and therefore they appear as radiolucent areas on a radiograph. The configuration of the pulp area is reduced with aging, in a few development abnormalities, or if the area is irritated. Dentin is deposited on the walls of the area as well during these processes. If there is irritation from decay or other trauma, the result is a condition called pulpitis. Pulpitis cannot generally be identified on a radiograph. Occasionally, there may be small areas with calcification in the pulp chamber that show up as radiopaque regions, but in general they have no clinical significance.

Acute apical periodontitis

Acute apical (or periapical) periodontitis, also known as AAP, is inflammation in the region of the periodontal ligament near the apex of the tooth. Clinically, the area is extremely painful, especially if tapped. Often, there is no change seen on a radiograph in the lamina dura or periodontal ligament spaces, although the latter may be wider than usual .There can be a variety of reasons for this inflammation. The most common causes are either some sort of irritation derived from pulpitis traveling via the root canal or response to some injury or foreign material (including restorations). If pulpitis is the causative agent, the damage is irreparable, the pulp tissue may be dead, and the pulp may need to be removed and a root canal procedure performed.

Acute apical abscess

If acute apical periodontitis caused by a dead tooth pulp is left untreated, an acute apical abscess (AAA) can develop. The area has become infected as evidenced by pus accumulated at the apex of the root, generalized pain and edema in the area, and pain and tenderness on percussion. Eventually, the tooth can come out of its socket and move around. The purulent exudate must be drained immediately to alleviate symptoms. On a radiograph, an early AAA may be difficult to pinpoint.

Changes to look for include an expansion of the periodontal ligament space. Advanced cases can show dark areas where the alveolar bone has been damaged.

Apical granuloma and treatments

When apical periodontitis becomes chronic, an apical granuloma may form as a mechanism to confine the irritants from the dead pulp and root canal. Essentially a fibrous pouch forms along the periodontal ligament around the chronically inflamed tissue in the apical area. Clinically, this sac formation relieves some of the pain and may arrest pustule formation, but generally root canal procedures are still necessary to prevent tooth loss. On a radiograph, an apical granuloma looks like a small dark rounded or oval area protruding from the apical area of the tooth. In the molar area of the upper jaw, this condition may cause the mucosal membranes of the sinus to become inflamed as well; this is known as antral mucositis.

Apical cyst is and how it is generally treated

When an apical granuloma expands in size, an apical cyst can form within the granuloma. The apical cyst consists of layers of squamous or scale-shaped epithelial cells that form a sac filled with liquid. Pressure builds up within the cyst and bone near the apex is resorbed. Clinically, the area may not hurt unless it has become infected. Nevertheless, all irritating substances in the dead pulp are generally eradicated and the root canal is closed up. Cysts are relatively easy to recognize on a radiograph because they appear as large radiolucent areas attached to the apex of the tooth and rimmed by a radiopaque outline of the bone.

Chronic apical abscess

A chronic apical abscess (CAA) is the end-result of a persistent acute apical abscess. It is often identified because a tooth is loose, or gum tissues are tender or swollen. As with the AAA, the pulp is dead and an infection is present in the apical area. A glaucomatous sac surrounds the purulent materials. There are two ways that chronic apical abscesses present themselves, and they are differentiated by the route for pus drainage. Most CAAs form canals or fistulas from the abscessed area through the alveolar bone to the outside of the gum where a boil or parulis is formed. Drainage of the CAA is generally then performed through this boil to alleviate the swelling and pain. On a radiograph, the fistula looks like a dark channel. Sometimes the chronic apical abscess does not form a fistula and the purulent material drains internally into the circulatory or lymphatic systems. For this type of CAA, the radiolucent sac has very indistinct borders indicating dispersion into other areas. In either type of CAA, a root canal procedure is indicated.

Apical condensing osteitis

Apical condensing osteitis (ACO) is dense bone formation in the apical tooth area that occurs in response to low-grade bacterial infection of the pulp. The alveolar bone is not actually destroyed in ACO. The condition is often asymptomatic but probing and other types of stimuli indicate that the pulp tissue is necrosed. On a radiograph, radiopaque areas are observed near the tooth apex. Condensing osteitis is prevalent in the premolar and molar regions of the mandible. As with other apical conditions, root canal treatment is generally performed in these patients.

Benign conditions in the apical region

Apical cementoma, also called periapical cementoma or cemental dysphasia, is a disorder in which connective tissues overgrow and destroy the lamina dura. The lesions themselves emanate from the periapical area, and appear dark on a radiograph with possible radiopaque infill containing cementum or bone during more advanced stages. Since pulp is not destroyed in this condition, the teeth are alive and no

root canal or other type of management is necessary. Another benign condition of the apical area is hypercementosis, in which excessive amounts of cementum deposit along the root of the tooth. On a radiograph, hypercementosis presents as either generalized enlargement of the root area or a nodule on the tip of the root.

Conditions in which the number of teeth is abnormal

There are a number of developmental aberrations in which the normal distribution or appearance of teeth is not seen. If the normal number of teeth is not observed, there are three possible conditions. In anodontia, either no teeth ever develop or the anomaly is acquired when all teeth are pulled out for some reason. People with anodontia are said to be edentulous. If one or more teeth or missing, the alteration is referred to as hypodontia; again this condition can be genetic or it can occur later. If many teeth are missing, the condition is sometimes referred to as oligodontia. If additional teeth are present, an inherited condition called hyperdontia exists. The extra teeth are also termed supernumerary.

Conditions in which the size of teeth is abnormal

Teeth can be bigger or smaller than expected. Relatively large dentition, termed macrodontia, is not very common. Pituitary giants experience generalized macrodontia, but other people may have individual teeth that are enlarged. Individuals with diminutive jaws appear to have macrodontia. Some people have microdontia in which all or some of the teeth are abnormally small relative to jaw size. The most common examples are small lateral incisors in the maxilla , a condition that tends to segregate in families, or small third molars. Microdontia is seen in pituitary dwarfs.

Shape and perceived number of teeth changed by division

There are several conditions where division or fusion errors give the appearance of abnormal dentition number. Two of these alterations are primarily observed in the front incisors. Gemination occurs when an individual tooth bud tries to split, but the division only occurs near the top. This gives the appearance of two teeth near the crown, but there is a common root canal. When two adjoining teeth join at the dentin and/or enamel areas, a process called fusion occurs. This condition reduces the total number of teeth observed, but a radiograph shows that there are actually two separate root canals.

Tooth shape or relationship changes enough to cause extraction

Adjacent teeth can join in the cementum region during root growth or eruption or occasionally later, and this phenomenon is known as concrescence. The most common sites for concrescence are various molars, particularly in the maxilla. The lack of separation and distorted relationship makes tooth extraction and corrective procedures very problematic in these teeth. Teeth can also be bent, particularly in the root area but sometimes in the crown. These curved shape changes are called dilacerations, and they can have a myriad of causes that are usually traumatic in nature. If a tooth is bent, the teeth in the area can be positioned incorrectly which again interferes with orthodontia or extraction.

Taurodontism and supernumerary roots

Both taurodontism and supernumerary roots are conditions in which the shape of root area of the tooth has developed abnormally. In taurodontism, the root is abbreviated and the pulp compartment is enlarged, given a squared-off appearance to the apical area. Supernumerary roots are additional roots on a tooth giving a branching appearance on a radiograph. Sometimes there are separate relatively small root canals in each branch as well. The number of branches is typically two or three. The periodontal ligament spaces can shift with supernumerary roots. This condition is most common in the canine and pre-molar regions of the lower jaw.

Enamel pearls

Enamel pearls are tiny spherical or oval pieces of enamel that adhere to the outside of the tooth. They are usually found in the molar region on the cervical neck of the tooth or in areas where branching has occurred. Since these pearls or enamelomas are made of enamel, they appear as opaque dots on a radiograph when observed in certain orientations that do not obscure them. Enamel pearls originating at branching points predispose an individual to periodontal disease if they are not removed because a pocket can form at the furcation. Enamel pearls can be confused radiographically with calcified areas in the pulp because both are radiopaque; the two can be distinguished by the fact that pulpal calcifications will be seen in various orientations whereas enamelomas will not.

Dens invaginatus and dens evaginatus

Dens invaginatus and dens evaginatus are both abnormalities in the pattern of the folding of the enamel at the occlusal surface. In dens invaginatus (also called dens in dente), the enamel on the crown folds inward leaving a hollow. This anomaly is relatively common. Since this invagination makes the pulp more vulnerable to exposure and the tooth more prone to decay, the crater is often closed up during youth. In dens evaginatus (also known as Leong's premolar), the enamel on the crown folds outward creating a bump. During dental probing, teeth with this type of elevation can be subjected to mechanical and inflammatory stresses so decay and pulp problems can occur here as well.

Enamel hypoplasia

Any condition in which the milieu of the enamel has been altered is called enamel hypoplasia. There are a number of possible manifestations of flawed enamel formation. If the alteration is localized to a single tooth as a pitted appearance, the causative agent was probably external trauma or infection. In baby teeth, this anomaly is often referred to as Turner's tooth. If a child is malnourished or contracts certain infections that produce a high fever, they can develop pitting or enamel hypoplasia on all or the majority of their teeth. This condition can develop in both primary incisors as well as permanent incisors if the deficiency or infection occurs during the first two years of life. Excessive exposure to fluorine can also produce another form of enamel hyperplasia in which the tooth surface appears mottled or discolored.

Amelogenesis imperfecta

If defective enamel formation or enamel hypoplasia is inherited, it is called amelogenesis imperfecta. Tooth decay is rare in individuals with this hereditary alteration. There are three types of amelogenesis imperfecta. In the first hypoplastic variation, the enamel's structure is unaltered but the width of its layer is very narrow. In the hypomineralized deviation, the concentration of minerals in the enamel is low which renders the tooth susceptible to pitting or splintering. The third variant is the hypomaturation type in which the grinding surface of the tooth has a white or pitted tip.

Dentinogenesis imperfecta

Dentinogenesis imperfecta is an inherited abnormality that involves the dentin and its connection with the enamel. The teeth have a shimmery appearance and they tend to crack. There are three classifications of dentinogenesis imperfecta differentiated primarily in terms of the association or lack thereof between generalized bone disease

and changes in the tooth structure. The first Type 1 occurs in individuals who also have generalized bone disease or osteogenesis imperfecta. In the other manifestations, this disorder only affects the teeth. Type 2 can be seen in the general population, whereas the more severe Type 3 occurs only in restricted populations in the eastern United States. On a radiograph, the pulp area looks destroyed and the roots are shortened and narrow with no evidence of a root canal.

Dental dysplasias

A dysplasia is some type of unusual growth or absence of a part. Two types of dysplasias are found in dentition. One is dentinal dysplasia in which the enamel appears normal but underneath the pulp and root areas are either defective or destroyed. Root development is minimal with this abnormality. In another type of dysphasia called regional odontodysplasia, both the dentin and enamel do not develop properly and the delineation between them disappears. Thus on a radiograph, the tooth is less radiopaque and has a ghost-like appearance. The pulp cavity also looks relatively large. Both of these conditions are uncommon.

Tooth defects

Tooth defects can be initiated through various types of mechanical or chemical wear and tear. Attrition and abrasion can look like tooth decay on a radiograph. Attrition is the wearing away of teeth by normal occlusal forces, whereas abrasion is wearing away by a mechanical device that has been introduced into the area. These mechanical devices include things like workplace items (for example, a hairdresser puts hairpins in her mouth), toothbrushes used incorrectly, ritual insertions into the oral cavity, and cocaine use. The abrasive pattern depends on the item used, but in all cases a radiolucent area is observed on a radiograph. Erosion or the chemical breakdown of the tooth's surface can also occur, possibly revealing the dentin underneath. Many of the causes involve

- 156 -

exposure to acids from medications or soda. Disorders of the digestive tract like bulimia or vomiting often lead to tooth erosion. On a radiograph, the crowns may look darker if erosion has occurred.

Tooth eruption abnormalities

Tooth eruption is the time period when the tooth emerges through the gum. If the tooth migrates or moves in a strange pattern prior to eruption, it will remain buried within the jaw bone. If the tooth moves after it has erupted, contact between normally adjacent teeth may be lost and this is referred to as drift. Teeth can also exchange normal positions upon eruption, a condition known as translocation. Translocation is usually not a major issue because no crowding or dental arch changes occur. On the other hand, sometimes a tooth can break out into an abnormal position. This situation, known as ectopic eruption, can create space problems and change the shape of the arch. Another condition, especially prevalent in the third molar region, is tooth impaction. Here, some spatial impedance such as another tooth changes the orientation of the imbedded tooth making eruption impossible; these teeth are usually extracted.

Appearance of fissural and dentigerous cysts

A cyst is any type of bone cavity lined with epithelial cells. Fissural cysts are sacs that emerge along embryonic junctures. There are three types of typical fissural cysts, each with a characteristic position. All look like radiolucent sacs on a radiograph. The nasopalatine cyst is typically located along the midline adjacent to the apices of incisors in the upper jaw. Further back along the midline, a median palatine cyst can occur. A globulomaxillary cyst is more elongated and is found between the lateral incisor and canine in the maxilla. A dentigerous cyst has a completely different origin; it occurs (usually in the third molar) when a tooth bud degenerates to form a cyst or sac. Again a dark sac is observed on a radiograph.

Appearance of cleft palate

A cleft is a narrow surface indentation that occurs because certain embryonic processes failed to fuse during development. In the context of dentistry, clefts can be found in the roof of the mouth, in either the bony front hard palate, the soft muscular palate located further back, or possibly in both. On a radiograph, the cleft area is radiolucent. Other developmental abnormalities can be found in conjunction with a cleft palate because the bones are shifted. Malpositioning is common as well as changes in the number of teeth ranging from complete anodontia to extra supernumerary dentition.

Classification of unknown lesion as benign or malignant

Areas that appear abnormal on a radiograph, but are not easily identified, can be tumors or cysts. A benign tumor is not cancerous, does not grow rapidly, and is usually not life-threatening. On a radiograph, a benign tumor presents as a dark, well-defined area. Other structures may be moved around on the radiograph, but they are not destroyed. Conversely, a malignant tumor is cancerous and fast-growing and it does participate in the destruction of other processes. Thus, on a radiograph, a malignant tumor is relatively radiolucent but generally more diffuse and the borders between the malignancy and other structures are less distinct. Tumors can also be radiopaque on the exposure if the density of the tumor tissue is higher than that in the type of cells it is infiltrating, for example bone or cartilage.

Fractures and embedded structures

Fractures to any part of the tooth appear as dark lines on a radiograph. If they occur in the crown area, they are easily recognizable. Cracks in the root area are more difficult to visualize because the alveolar bone is also in the area. Identification of fractures is important, because pulp damage can lead to other undesirable pathology. Most foreign bodies like implants contain metal are readily identifiable because they are very radiopaque. Root tips can sometimes be embedded within the jaw and should be removed; they can be found by looking for their canal or their funnel-like shape.

Salivary stones

Calcifications or salivary stones can occur in the soft tissues of the salivary glands and associated ducts. They can predispose an individual to infection, edema, and obstruction. Thus, even though they do not directly affect the teeth, salivary stones are in the general area and do have diagnostic significance. The stones are easily visualized on radiographs as intensely radiopaque spots. Because of their position, salivary stones are usually identified on occlusal or panoramic films, although they can sometimes be seen on periapical exposures. Salivary stones can also be visualized by injecting radiopaque media into the salivary ducts and glands, a technique called sialography.

Legal Considerations

Governing dental equipment in a dental office

Use of various types of dental equipment must meet official federal performance standards. Radiation standards are generally also established locally by the city, county and/or state. In particular, radiation inspections are usually required 2 or 3 times a year. In terms of professional licensure for radiation use, states generally set their own guidelines. A dental hygienist is a licensed specialist, but additional certification in radiography may or may not be obligatory. A dental assistant may be expected to take an examination related to radiology if they take radiographs. For both types of professionals, some states only require general supervision by or presence of a dentist.

Concept of respondent superior

The concept of respondent superior is a legal doctrine placing professional and legal liability with the supervising professional. In other words, in a dental practice, the dentist accepts responsibility for the actions of other professionals like dental hygienists or assistants. A hygienist or assistant under the employ of the dentist is not ultimately responsible, but they could be expected to accept some of the financial burden if found negligent. Therefore, liability insurance is still necessary. An independent contractor can be found responsible and can be sued. In addition, negative input in the office setting can be used as legal evidence of negligence.

Components of informed consent

Dental and medical professionals must obtain informed consent from a patient or their representative (such as the parent or guardian) before initiating procedures. Informed consent involves a complete explanation or full disclosure of the process including its rationale, its benefits, and the possible negative consequences. In the dental office, informed consent should be obtained before performing radiography. If informed consent is denied, the radiograph cannot be taken and an essential part of the diagnostic process is lost.

Dental records, ownership and retention parameters

Dental records including radiographs are legal documents. Therefore, dates, number and types of radiographic procedures must be immediately entered. The radiographs themselves must also be tagged and dated and securely fastened to the chart. All parts of the record are confidential and are considered to be owned by the dentist. The latter means that the dentist is not allowed to give the radiographs to the patient or insurance company, although rules pertaining to distribution of duplicates vary by locality. The minimum period for record retention is 6 or 7 years (depending on local legislation) after the individual stops their association with the dental office.

Privacy standards section of the Health Insurance Portability and Accountability Act of 1996

The HIPAA or the Health Insurance Portability and Accountability Act of 1996 has three sections: (1) privacy standards, (2) patients' rights, and (3) administrative requirements. The Act requires electronic standardization of patient health care data. The privacy standards section deals primarily with protected health information or PHI. It requires the professional to obtain authorization from the patient before health information can be disclosed for treatment, payment, or healthcare related procedures. This can be in the form of written consent or they can sign an Acknowledgment of Receipt Notice of Privacy Practices. There are only a few exceptions to these requirements such possible child abuse. Non-adherence can result in civil penalties, fines, or criminal punishments.

Nature of the patients' rights section of the HIPAA

The patients' rights section of the HIPAA deals with the entitlements of patients or their representative to obtain their health information. The essence of patients' rights is that they can look at their records, copy them, question violations of rules, and request non-electronic forms of transmission. For minors, these rights generally apply to their parents unless there has been another legal edict. In addition, if the healthcare or dental professional wants to release any information for reason besides treatment, payment, or operations, they must inform the patient.

Administrative requirement section of the HIPAA

The administrative requirements section of the HIPAA mandates that dental offices have a written privacy policy which can be distributed to the patient. It also requires the dentist to train and familiarize the other personnel in details of the privacy policy and means of documentation. This section also compels the dentist to appoint an office privacy officer to monitor these policies, and another individual to handle complaints. A Notice of Privacy Practices must be in place. If third parties are to have access to patient information, they must be clearly acknowledged as well.

Managing patients with special needs

A good chair side manner is paramount in dealing with any patient. The major physical disability that might pose a problem is a patient's inability to control movement as in certain spastic disorders; here a friend wearing protective gear should assist and steady the patient, not the dental professional. Individuals with developmental disabilities are usually harder to manage, and use of sedatives or anesthesia may be necessary. Most types of radiographs can be done without moving an immobile patient out of a wheelchair, and if they are confined to their beds or home, there are mobile x-ray units available. Alternative methods of communication need to be continually reinforced for hearing or vision impaired individuals.

Pediatric patients and ways to manage issues

Pediatric patients may be unfamiliar with the process of having x-rays taken, so any attempt to explain or show them what will occur during the exposure is helpful. One of the major management issues is getting the pediatric patient to understand that they must remain perfectly still when the shot is being taken. In addition, some children cannot endure certain types of film placements. Since their mouth is smaller than that of an adult, more latitude can be allowed in the technique or placement of the film. For example, an acceptable exposure can be taken by having the child bite down on a periapical film while the operator increases the vertical angulation. Reverse bitewings are often done on pediatric patients because they tend to dislodge regular bitewings; in the reverse technique the bitewing is positioned near the cheek and the exposure is taken as a lateral oblique view from the opposite side. Occasionally, extraoral films are done instead.

Special Problems

Unconventional radiographic methods required to localize structures

There are 4 methods of defining the relationship between different structures in the oral cavity. In the first method, two objects are localized by definition on a normal radiograph. In other words, the more defined object is considered to be located lingually on the tongue side because that is the position of the film. The tube shift approach compares two radiographs whose only difference is a slight shift of the x-ray tube's horizontal angulation. Here a principle called the buccal-object rule is employed; according to this rule, buccal objects appear to move in the opposite direction. These techniques are also employed to localize foreign objects or unerupted teeth. A similar type of relationship can be found when observing some older pantomographic exposures. Periapical films used in conjunction with occlusal films taken at right angles can provide information about structural relationships as well.

Techniques to get better exposures of the third molars

It is difficult to get good exposures of third molars, and often extraoral or panoramic views must be taken. The major problem with normal intraoral exposures of the upper jaw is excitation of the gag reflex. A hemostat is generally used to keep the film away from the palate and vertical angulation is increased to minimize spatial errors. In the mandible, it is very hard to place the film far enough back in the mouth so techniques to relax the muscle on the floor of the mouth, move the tongue to the side, and/or direct the beam from the distal side are usually employed.

Developmental abnormalities that can affect film placement

If an individual has a narrow dental arch, it may be necessary to use smaller #0 or #1 films for exposures of the front of the mouth. If the patient has a shallow palatial vault, it may be difficult to place the film in the correct position using the paralleling method; solutions include use of a smaller film size or the bisecting technique. Some people have stiff lingual tongue attachments which make it difficult to place a film packet on the floor of the mouth; here the bisecting-angle technique is generally used. If a patient has a bony ridge or torus in the mandible, the film packet must be put over it and the vertical angulation must be augmented to balance the larger angle between the film and the long axis of the tooth. Presence of an oversized palatial cusp at the first premolar of the maxilla is a widespread abnormality; in these cases, the canine will appear to be overlapped unless the direction of the x-ray beam is more distal.

Trismus and radiographs

Patients with infections or some type of injury may be unable to open their mouth to some extent, a condition called trismus. Diagnostic radiographs are usually indicated in these individuals. If possible, intraoral exposures can be taken by inserting the film with a hemostat, orienting it correctly after insertion, and instructing the patient to hold the hemostat. If intraoral films cannot be successfully attempted, then panoramic or extraoral techniques can be employed. Good operator chairside technique is crucial for problems like these.

Successful radiographs in patients with endodontic problems

Individuals undergoing management of endodontic or pulp problems usually have rubber dams in the oral cavity. The best way to take a radiograph is to remove the frame of the dam and arrange the film packet by using a hemostat or Snap-a-Ray holder. The patient holds the film-holder in an orientation parallel to the tooth. The shot should be taken very quickly. Several types of radiopaque products that aid visualization may be used in conjunction with the radiograph. These include intraoral grids placed on the film packet or injection of radiopaque media into certain areas.

Secret Key #1 - Time is Your Greatest Enemy

Pace Yourself

Wear a watch. At the beginning of the test, check the time (or start a chronometer on your watch to count the minutes), and check the time after every few questions to make sure you are "on schedule."

If you are forced to speed up, do it efficiently. Usually one or more answer choices can be eliminated without too much difficulty. Above all, don't panic. Don't speed up and just begin guessing at random choices. By pacing yourself, and continually monitoring your progress against your watch, you will always know exactly how far ahead or behind you are with your available time. If you find that you are one minute behind on the test, don't skip one question without spending any time on it, just to catch back up. Take 15 fewer seconds on the next four questions, and after four questions you'll have caught back up. Once you catch back up, you can continue working each problem at your normal pace.

Furthermore, don't dwell on the problems that you were rushed on. If a problem was taking up too much time and you made a hurried guess, it must be difficult. The difficult questions are the ones you are most likely to miss anyway, so it isn't a big loss. It is better to end with more time than you need than to run out of time.

Lastly, sometimes it is beneficial to slow down if you are constantly getting ahead of time. You are always more likely to catch a careless mistake by working more slowly than quickly, and among very high-scoring test takers (those who are likely to have lots of time left over), careless errors affect the score more than mastery of material.

Secret Key #2 - Guessing is not Guesswork

You probably know that guessing is a good idea - unlike other standardized tests, there is no penalty for getting a wrong answer. Even if you have no idea about a question, you still have a 20-25% chance of getting it right.

Most test takers do not understand the impact that proper guessing can have on their score. Unless you score extremely high, guessing will significantly contribute to your final score.

Monkeys Take the Test

What most test takers don't realize is that to insure that 20-25% chance, you have to guess randomly. If you put 20 monkeys in a room to take this test, assuming they answered once per question and behaved themselves, on average they would get 20-25% of the questions correct. Put 20 test takers in the room, and the average will be much lower among guessed questions. Why?

1. The test writers intentionally writes deceptive answer choices that "look" right. A test taker has no idea about a question, so picks the "best looking" answer, which is often wrong. The monkey has no idea what looks good and what doesn't, so will consistently be lucky about 20-25% of the time.

2. Test takers will eliminate answer choices from the guessing pool based on a hunch or intuition. Simple but correct answers often get excluded, leaving a 0% chance of being correct. The monkey has no clue, and often gets lucky with the best choice.

This is why the process of elimination endorsed by most test courses is flawed and detrimental to your performance- test takers don't guess, they make an ignorant stab in the dark that is usually worse than random.

$5 Challenge

Let me introduce one of the most valuable ideas of this course- the $5 challenge:

You only mark your "best guess" if you are willing to bet $5 on it.
You only eliminate choices from guessing if you are willing to bet $5 on it.

Why $5? Five dollars is an amount of money that is small yet not insignificant, and can really add up fast (20 questions could cost you $100). Likewise, each answer choice on one question of the test will have a small impact on your overall score, but it can really add up to a lot of points in the end.

The process of elimination IS valuable. The following shows your chance of guessing it right:

If you eliminate wrong answer choices until only this many answer choices remain:	1	2	3
Chance of getting it correct:	100%	50%	33%

However, if you accidentally eliminate the right answer or go on a hunch for an incorrect answer, your chances drop dramatically: to 0%. By guessing among all the answer choices, you are GUARANTEED to have a shot at the right answer.

That's why the $5 test is so valuable- if you give up the advantage and safety of a pure guess, it had better be worth the risk.

What we still haven't covered is how to be sure that whatever guess you make is truly random. Here's the easiest way:

Always pick the first answer choice among those remaining.

Such a technique means that you have decided, **before you see a single test question**, exactly how you are going to guess- and since the order of choices tells you nothing about which one is correct, this guessing technique is perfectly random. This section is not meant to scare you away from making educated guesses or eliminating choices- you just need to define when a choice is worth eliminating. The $5 test, along with a pre-defined random guessing strategy, is the best way to make sure you reap all of the benefits of guessing.

Secret Key #3 - Practice Smarter, Not Harder

Many test takers delay the test preparation process because they dread the awful amounts of practice time they think necessary to succeed on the test. We have refined an effective method that will take you only a fraction of the time.

There are a number of "obstacles" in your way to succeed. Among these are answering questions, finishing in time, and mastering test-taking strategies. All must be executed on the day of the test at peak performance, or your score will suffer. The test is a mental marathon that has a large impact on your future.

Just like a marathon runner, it is important to work your way up to the full challenge. So first you just worry about questions, and then time, and finally strategy:

Success Strategy

1. Find a good source for practice tests.
2. If you are willing to make a larger time investment, consider using more than one study guide- often the different approaches of multiple authors will help you "get" difficult

concepts.

3. Take a practice test with no time constraints, with all study helps "open book." Take your time with questions and focus on applying strategies.
4. Take a practice test with time constraints, with all guides "open book."
5. Take a final practice test with no open material and time limits

If you have time to take more practice tests, just repeat step 5. By gradually exposing yourself to the full rigors of the test environment, you will condition your mind to the stress of test day and maximize your success.

Secret Key #4 - Prepare, Don't Procrastinate

Let me state an obvious fact: if you take the test three times, you will get three different scores. This is due to the way you feel on test day, the level of preparedness you have, and, despite the test writers' claims to the contrary, some tests WILL be easier for you than others.

Since your future depends so much on your score, you should maximize your chances of success. In order to maximize the likelihood of success, you've got to prepare in advance. This means taking practice tests and spending time learning the information and test taking strategies you will need to succeed.

Never take the test as a "practice" test, expecting that you can just take it again if you need to. Feel free to take sample tests on your own, but when you go to take the official test, be prepared, be focused, and do your best the first time!

Secret Key #5 - Test Yourself

Everyone knows that time is money. There is no need to spend too much of your time or too little of your time preparing for the test. You should only spend as much of your precious time preparing as is necessary for you to get the score you need.

Once you have taken a practice test under real conditions of time constraints, then you will know if you are ready for the test or not. If you have scored extremely high the first time that you take the practice test, then there is not much point in spending countless hours studying. You are already there.

Benchmark your abilities by retaking practice tests and seeing how much you have improved. Once you score high enough to guarantee success, then you are ready.

If you have scored well below where you need, then knuckle down and begin studying in earnest. Check your improvement regularly through the use of practice tests under real conditions. Above all, don't worry, panic, or give up. The key is perseverance!

Then, when you go to take the test, remain confident and remember how well you did on the practice tests. If you can score high enough on a practice test, then you can do the same on the real thing.

General Strategies

The most important thing you can do is to ignore your fears and jump into the test immediately- do not be overwhelmed by any strange-sounding terms. You have to jump into the test like jumping into a pool- all at once is the easiest way.

Make Predictions

As you read and understand the question, try to guess what the answer will be. Remember that several of the answer choices are wrong, and once you begin reading them, your mind will immediately become cluttered with answer choices designed to throw you off. Your mind is typically the most focused immediately after you have read the question and digested its contents. If you can, try to predict what the correct answer will be. You may be surprised at what you can predict.

Quickly scan the choices and see if your prediction is in the listed answer choices. If it is, then you can be quite confident that you have the right answer. It still won't hurt to check the other answer choices, but most of the time, you've got it!

Answer the Question

It may seem obvious to only pick answer choices that answer the question, but the test writers can create some excellent answer choices that are wrong. Don't pick an answer just because it sounds right, or you believe it to be true. It MUST answer the question. Once you've made your selection, always go back and check it against the question and make sure that you didn't misread the question, and the answer choice does answer the question posed.

Benchmark

After you read the first answer choice, decide if you think it sounds correct or not. If it doesn't, move on to the next answer choice. If it does, mentally mark that answer choice.

This doesn't mean that you've definitely selected it as your answer choice, it just means that it's the best you've seen thus far. Go ahead and read the next choice. If the next choice is worse than the one you've already selected, keep going to the next answer choice. If the next choice is better than the choice you've already selected, mentally mark the new answer choice as your best guess.

The first answer choice that you select becomes your standard. Every other answer choice must be benchmarked against that standard. That choice is correct until proven otherwise by another answer choice beating it out. Once you've decided that no other answer choice seems as good, do one final check to ensure that your answer choice answers the question posed.

Valid Information

Don't discount any of the information provided in the question. Every piece of information may be necessary to determine the correct answer. None of the information in the question is there to throw you off (while the answer choices will certainly have information to throw you off). If two seemingly unrelated topics are discussed, don't ignore either. You can be confident there is a relationship, or it wouldn't be included in the question, and you are probably going to have to determine what is that relationship to find the answer.

Avoid "Fact Traps"

Don't get distracted by a choice that is factually true. Your search is for the answer that answers the question. Stay focused and don't fall for an answer that is true but incorrect. Always go back to the question and make sure you're choosing an answer that actually answers the question and is not just a true statement. An answer can be factually correct, but it MUST answer the question asked. Additionally, two answers can both be seemingly correct, so be sure to read all of the answer choices, and make sure that you get the one that BEST answers the question.

Milk the Question

Some of the questions may throw you completely off. They might deal with a subject you have not been exposed to, or one that you haven't reviewed in years. While your lack of knowledge about the subject will be a hindrance, the question itself can give you many clues that will help you find the correct answer. Read the question carefully and look for clues. Watch particularly for adjectives and nouns describing difficult terms or words that you don't recognize. Regardless of if you completely understand a word or not, replacing it with a synonym either provided or one you more familiar with may help you to understand what the questions are asking. Rather than wracking your mind about specific detailed information concerning a difficult term or word, try to use mental substitutes that are easier to understand.

The Trap of Familiarity

Don't just choose a word because you recognize it. On difficult questions, you may not recognize a number of words in the answer choices. The test writers don't put "make-believe" words on the test; so don't think that just because you only recognize all the words in one answer choice means that answer choice must be correct. If you only recognize words in one answer choice, then focus on that one. Is it correct? Try your best to determine if it is correct. If it is, that is great, but if it doesn't, eliminate it. Each word and answer choice you eliminate increases your chances of getting the question correct, even if you then have to guess among the unfamiliar choices.

Eliminate Answers

Eliminate choices as soon as you realize they are wrong. But be careful! Make sure you consider all of the possible answer choices. Just because one appears right, doesn't mean that the next one won't be even better! The test writers will usually put more than one good answer choice for every question, so read all of them. Don't worry if you are stuck between two that seem right. By getting down to just two remaining possible choices, your odds are now 50/50. Rather than wasting too much time, play the odds. You are guessing, but guessing wisely, because you've been able to knock out some of the answer choices that you know are wrong. If you are eliminating choices and realize that the last answer choice you are left with is also obviously wrong, don't panic. Start over and consider each choice again. There may easily be something that you missed the first time and will realize on the second pass.

Tough Questions

If you are stumped on a problem or it appears too hard or too difficult, don't waste time. Move on! Remember though, if you can quickly check for obviously incorrect answer choices, your chances of guessing correctly are greatly improved. Before you completely give up, at least try to knock out a couple of possible answers. Eliminate what you can and then guess at the remaining answer choices before moving on.

Brainstorm

If you get stuck on a difficult question, spend a few seconds quickly brainstorming. Run through the complete list of possible answer choices. Look at each choice and ask yourself, "Could this answer the question satisfactorily?" Go through each answer choice and consider it independently of the other. By systematically going through all possibilities, you may find something that you would otherwise overlook. Remember that when you get stuck, it's important to try to keep moving.

Read Carefully

Understand the problem. Read the question and answer choices carefully. Don't miss the question because you misread the terms. You have plenty of time to read each question thoroughly and make sure you understand what is being asked. Yet a happy medium must be attained, so don't waste too much time. You must read carefully, but efficiently.

Face Value

When in doubt, use common sense. Always accept the situation in the problem at face value. Don't read too much into it. These problems will not require you to make huge leaps of logic. The test writers aren't trying to throw you off with a cheap trick. If you have to go beyond creativity and make a leap of logic in order to have an answer choice answer the question, then you should look at the other answer choices. Don't overcomplicate the problem by creating theoretical relationships or explanations that will warp time or space. These are normal problems rooted in reality. It's just that the applicable relationship or explanation may not be readily apparent and you have to figure things out. Use your common sense to interpret anything that isn't clear.

Prefixes

If you're having trouble with a word in the question or answer choices, try dissecting it. Take advantage of every clue that the word might include. Prefixes and suffixes can be a huge help. Usually they allow you to determine a basic meaning. Pre- means before, post- means after, pro - is positive, de- is negative. From these prefixes and suffixes, you can get an idea of the general meaning of the word and try to put it into context. Beware though of any traps. Just because con is the opposite of pro, doesn't necessarily mean congress is the opposite of progress!

Hedge Phrases

Watch out for critical "hedge" phrases, such as likely, may, can, will often, sometimes, often, almost, mostly, usually, generally, rarely, sometimes. Question writers insert these hedge phrases to cover every possibility. Often an answer choice will be wrong simply because it leaves no room for exception. Avoid answer choices that have definitive words like "exactly," and "always".

Switchback Words

Stay alert for "switchbacks". These are the words and phrases frequently used to alert you to shifts in thought. The most common switchback word is "but". Others include although, however, nevertheless, on the other hand, even though, while, in spite of, despite, regardless of.

New Information

Correct answer choices will rarely have completely new information included. Answer choices typically are straightforward reflections of the material asked about and will directly relate to the question. If a new piece of information is included in an answer choice that doesn't even seem to relate to the topic being asked about, then that answer choice is likely incorrect. All of the information needed to answer the question is usually provided for you, and so you should not have to make guesses that are unsupported or choose answer choices that require unknown information that cannot be reasoned on its own.

Time Management

On technical questions, don't get lost on the technical terms. Don't spend too much time on any one question. If you don't know what a term means, then since you don't have a dictionary, odds are you aren't going to get much further. You should immediately recognize terms as whether or not you know them. If you don't, work with the other clues that you have, the other answer choices and terms provided, but don't waste too much time trying to figure out a difficult term.

Contextual Clues

Look for contextual clues. An answer can be right but not correct. The contextual clues will help you find the answer that is most right and is correct. Understand the context in which a phrase or statement is made. This will help you make important distinctions.

Don't Panic

Panicking will not answer any questions for you. Therefore, it isn't helpful. When you first see the question, if your mind goes blank, take a deep breath. Force yourself to mechanically go through the steps of solving the problem and using the strategies you've learned.

Pace Yourself

Don't get clock fever. It's easy to be overwhelmed when you're looking at a page full of questions, your mind is full of random thoughts and feeling confused, and the clock is ticking down faster than you would like. Calm down and maintain the pace that you have set for yourself. As long as you are on track by monitoring your pace, you are guaranteed to have enough time for yourself. When you get to the last few minutes of the test, it may seem like you won't have enough time left, but if you only have as many questions as you should have left at that point, then you're right on track!

Answer Selection

The best way to pick an answer choice is to eliminate all of those that are wrong, until only one is left and confirm that is the correct answer. Sometimes though, an answer choice may immediately look right. Be careful! Take a second to make sure that the other choices are not equally obvious. Don't make a hasty mistake. There are only two times that you should stop before checking other answers. First is when you are positive that the answer choice you have selected is correct. Second is when time is almost out and you have to make a quick guess!

Check Your Work

Since you will probably not know every term listed and the answer to every question, it is important that you get credit for the ones that you do know. Don't miss any questions through careless mistakes. If at all possible, try to take a second to look back over your answer selection and make sure you've selected the correct answer choice and haven't made a costly careless mistake (such as marking an answer choice that you didn't mean to mark). This quick double check should more than pay for itself in caught mistakes for the time it costs.

Beware of Directly Quoted Answers

Sometimes an answer choice will repeat word for word a portion of the question or reference section. However, beware of such exact duplication – it may be a trap! More than likely, the correct choice will paraphrase or summarize a point, rather than being exactly the same wording.

Slang

Scientific sounding answers are better than slang ones. An answer choice that begins "To compare the outcomes…" is much more likely to be correct than one that begins "Because some people insisted…"

Extreme Statements

Avoid wild answers that throw out highly controversial ideas that are proclaimed as established fact. An answer choice that states the "process should be used in certain situations, if…" is much more likely to be correct than one that states the "process should be discontinued completely." The first is a calm rational statement and doesn't even make a definitive, uncompromising stance, using a hedge word "if" to provide wiggle room, whereas the second choice is a radical idea and far more extreme.

Answer Choice Families

When you have two or more answer choices that are direct opposites or parallels, one of them is usually the correct answer. For instance, if one answer choice states "x increases" and another answer choice states "x decreases" or "y increases," then those two or three answer choices are very similar in construction and fall into the same family of answer choices. A family of answer choices is when two or three answer choices are very similar in construction, and yet often have a directly opposite meaning. Usually the correct answer choice will be in that family of answer choices. The "odd man out" or answer choice that doesn't seem to fit the parallel construction of the other answer choices is more likely to be incorrect.

Special Report: Additional Bonus Material

Due to our efforts to try to keep this book to a manageable length, we've created a link that will give you access to all of your additional bonus material.

Please visit http://www.mometrix.com/bonus948/danbcda to access the information.